D1563923

BOTANICAL MIXED DRINKS RECIPE BOOK

Published by Herbal Academy
24 South Road, Bedford, MA 01731
Copyright © 2023 Herbal Academy

theherbalacademy.com

Text © 2023 Herbal Academy

Book Design:
Amber Meyers, Cover Design, Interior Design
Emay Allmendinger, Botanical Illustrator, Interior Design

Editors:
Jane Metzger, M.S.
Lisa Olson, RH(AHG)
Meagan Visser, BSN

Recipe Contributors:
Amber Meyers
Catarina Seixas
Cristina Asensio-Foley
Hannah Lasorsa
Heather Skasick
Heather Wood Buzzard
Holly Hutton, RH(AHG)
Jane Metzger, M.S.
Jill York
Lisa Olson, RH(AHG)
Meagan Visser, BSN
Safiyyah Bazemore
Sarah Baldwin
Stacy Karen

International Standard Book Number
978-1-950671-04-5

Botanical
MIXED DRINKS
Recipe Book

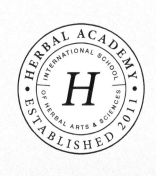
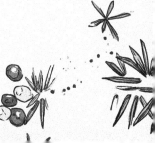

PRAISE FOR THE BOOK

"*Botanical beverages can be some of the simplest ways to engage our senses and experience the wealth of plants for fun. health. and wellbeing. Whether it's for a season of the year or a favorite ingredient. the Botanical Mixed Drinks Recipe Book gives you the inspiration to create something wonderful and delicious.*"

    — **BEVIN CLARE**, L.D.N., M.S., R.H., Professor, Herbalist, and Nutritionist at the Maryland University of Integrative Health and Author of *Spice Apothecary*

"*What herbal enthusiast doesn't love to put together a delicious botanical cocktail or mocktail to impress friends and family? I have been looking for new inspiration for my drinks cabinet for a while now—and I've just found it! With their gorgeous signature style. packed full of wonderful recipes and tips. this is my new go-to guide. Cheers!*"

    — **PAMELA SPENCE**, M.A. (Hons), B.Sc. (Hons), M.N.I.M.H., Medical Herbalist

"*From Elderflower Champagne to Lemon Balm Martinis. in* Botanical Mixed Drinks Recipe Book. *Herbal Academy has put together a comprehensive and easy to use recipe book to supercharge your cocktails into dazzling drinks full of herbs and spices. I love how the festive drinks are categorized by season and the focus on cocktails and mocktails alike. There is something here for everyone! This delightful resource full of intriguing herbal infused drinks will bring new meaning and enthusiasm to the word 'cheers'!*"

    — **KAMI MCBRIDE**, Author of *The Herbal Kitchen* and teacher of herbal medicine since 1988

TABLE OF
CONTENTS

PRAISE FOR THE BOOK

"*The Herbal Academy team assembled this delightful book to inspire you in your herbal journey through the joyful and experiential lens of botanical cocktails. As someone who really enjoys approaching herbs and the kitchen in a seasonal manner, I especially like the way the book was assembled by season—each recipe adorned with gorgeous artwork that captures the vibe of the cocktail and entices you to help you decide which drink to whip up next. This is the perfect book to help make your next gathering extra special or simply to embody and celebrate each season with a classy, unique herbal drink.*"

— **MARIA NOËL GROVES**, RH (AHG), Clinical Herbalist and Author of *Body into Balance* and *Grow Your Own Herbal Remedies*

"*The Botanical Mixed Drinks Recipe Book is a wonderful guide for making your own cocktails and mocktails with herbs, flowers, and plants. This book will definitely be one that I turn to time and time again to make up beautifully crafted drinks for celebrations big and small!*"

— **COLLEEN CODEKAS**, Author of *Healing Herbal Infusions* and blogger at Grow Forage Cook Ferment

"*Herbal Academy's Botanical Mixed Drinks Recipe Book is truly inspired in its creativity and inventive way of incorporating plants into your everyday. While it is deeply rooted in its herbal foundations, I adore the step by step instructions, the fun, delicious beverages mixed from its pages will have you wanting more.*"

— **ALYSON MORGAN**, Author of *Our Kindred Home*

ACKNOWLEDGMENTS

With our penchant for soothing herbal teas, refreshing botanical shrubs, warming winter cocoas, and tasty before-dinner apéritifs, you could say herbalists know drinks. Caught a chill? Mix up a gingery hot toddy. Feeling hot? Have a quenching citrus agua fresca. Nursing a cold? Brew up an immune-boosting cup of tea. Need a mental boost? Pep it up with a rosemary tonic. Botanical drinks are one of the ways we enjoy the benefits of plants, express our herbal creativity, and offer hospitality and health to loved ones, guests, and our herbal community.

The *Botanical Mixed Drinks Recipe Book* is the second installment in our Herbal Academy Recipe Book Collection and an extension of our online **Botanical Mixed Drinks Workshop**. We, as an Herbal Academy team, have come together, putting to paper an array of recipes that incorporate our favorite herbs and flavors and reflect the moods and needs of each season. We drew inspiration from our personal experiences working with herbs, some of our most-cherished recipes we use in our own homes, and recipe foundations we share within our classroom walls. This fusion of inspiration turned recipe creation required a full Herbal Academy collaborative production, requiring many afternoon happy hours (and mocktail hours!) of delicious taste-testing sessions! We happily obliged.

The original **Botanical Mixed Drinks Workshop** we offered online ultimately blossomed into this larger collection of recipes developed and polished by the Herbal Academy team of Meagan Visser, Lisa Olson, Jane Metzger, and Amber Meyers with support from recipe contributors and testers Cristina Asensio-Foley, Sarah Baldwin, Safiyyah Bazemore, Heather Wood Buzzard, Holly Hutton, Stacy Karen, Hannah Lasorsa, Catarina Seixas, Heather Skasick, and Jill York. Botanical illustrator Emay Allmendinger teamed up with Amber Meyers to bring the book's visual presentation to life with a gorgeous design and whimsical illustrations.

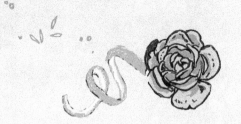

As with any Herbal Academy project, this book is the result of a multifaceted team collaboration that pulls inspiration and innovation from many, and a powerhouse group to support the creative process, and so we express gratitude for the entire group of Herbal Academy team members that have also contributed to this success! We also toast to our many friends and family members who gathered with us for a sip and experienced this festive journey along with us, which honors the community-centered intention behind this botanical mixology creation.

This book wouldn't be complete without a special mention for Herbal Academy Founder Marlene Adelmann, who was a lover of herbalism and a consummate host who always went the extra mile to offer a welcoming cup of tea, an herbal kombucha, or a creative botanical drink to coworkers, friends, family, and guests. It is in that spirit that we extend this heartfully crafted, carefully curated collection of festive recipes to you.

Cheers!

JANE METZGER AND AMBER MEYERS
CO-DIRECTORS, HERBAL ACADEMY

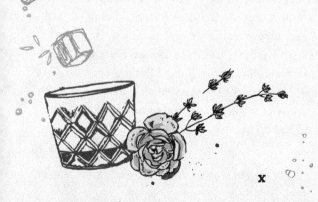

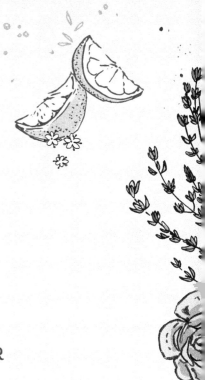

DISCLAIMER

While the herbs selected for these recipes are typically safe in the suggested amounts for the general population, always research the safety of individual herbs in the case of particular health conditions.

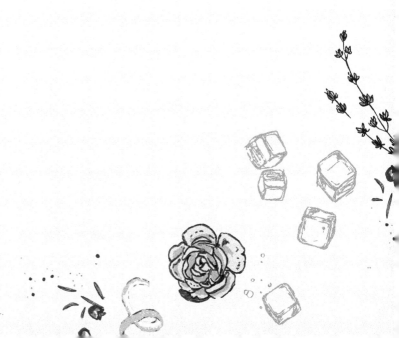

CHAPTER ONE

WELCOME!

Since time immemorial, people have come together to celebrate the joys of life—from the changing of the seasons to the birth of a new family member. One common thread woven throughout so many of these festivities is the presence of celebratory drinks made with botanicals, including seasonal fruits, herbs, and spices— and for some occasions—spirits!

Herbalists (and herb-curious folks) are especially well-equipped for making festive drinks because our kitchens are often already stocked with floral syrups, herbal bitters, infused vinegars, and other ingredients that are a practical choice for capturing the botanical goodness and benefits of plants. For those that enjoy hand-crafted mixed drinks from time to time, these herbal preparations can elevate drink recipes from good to great. In turn, a well-crafted drink can be an appealing way to incorporate more botanicals into the occasional alcoholic (or non-alcoholic) beverage and celebrate seasonal rhythms and harvests.

If you don't already have these foundational preparations, don't worry—we'll cover step-by-step instructions for creating a well-stocked herbal bar with 12 foundational recipes to get you started. We're also sharing 82 uniquely creative botanical mixed drink recipes that will give you plenty of inspiration all year long, plus a helpful checklist and tables to make serving up your own botanical cocktails and mocktails as easy as possible.

All of the recipes featured throughout this book include herbs and spices that can support your health and tantalize your taste buds—from peppermint and rose to cinnamon and cardamom. You can find these ingredients at your local grocery store, in your garden, or online, and—for the adventurous mixologist—you can even forage some of the ingredients in the forests, meadows, and wild spaces near your home. The recipes are organized by season to help you tune into seasonal rhythms, encouraging the use of herbs and fruits at their peak freshness and utilizing their energetics to bring balance to the body during summer's heat, winter's chill, and other seasonal shifts.

The flavors of these mixed drinks range from sweet to sour with an array of botanical accents. You'll find cocktail recipes with options for non-alcoholic substitutions as well as straight-up mocktails highlighting botanical ingredients. Depending on their ingredients, these drinks are often enjoyed at various times of the day; there are certain drinks for morning and brunch, drinks enjoyed with meals, pre- and post-meal apéritifs and digestifs, and even nightcaps to sip before bed.

While we don't advise partaking in alcoholic drinks frequently—these beverages are best enjoyed on occasion—it's fun to note how versatile both cocktails and mocktails are as yet another way to integrate herbs into your life.

Herbal Cheers!
THE HERBAL ACADEMY TEAM

Creating a
MIXED DRINKS PANTRY

When gathering supplies to create mixed drinks, things can get fancy (and expensive) quickly! However, we like to keep things as straightforward as possible by using supplies most of us already have around our home or items that are easy to purchase in local stores or thrift shops.

Botanical Mixed Drinks Supply Checklist

KITCHEN EQUIPMENT

- [ ] Glass canning jars with lids
- [ ] Fine-mesh sieves
- [ ] Spoons
- [ ] Measuring cups and spoons
- [ ] Bowls and small plates
- [ ] Cocktail picks or skewers
- [ ] Vegetable peeler
- [ ] Coffee filters
- [ ] Natural waxed paper
- [ ] Blender
- [ ] Coffee grinder
- [ ] Saucepans

GLASSWARE

- [ ] Champagne flute glasses
- [ ] Collins/highball glasses
- [ ] Cordial glasses
- [ ] Coupe glasses
- [ ] Heatproof mugs
- [ ] Martini glasses
- [ ] Old-fashioned/rocks glasses
- [ ] Punch glasses
- [ ] Wine/snifter glasses

APOTHECARY EQUIPMENT

- [ ] Boston round amber bottles with lids
- [ ] Bottle labels
- [ ] Mortar and pestle
- [ ] Pipette
- [ ] Small funnel

DRINK INGREDIENTS

- [ ] Base spirits (e.g., bourbon, brandy, gin, rum, scotch, vodka)
- [ ] Botanicals
- [ ] Carbonated water
- [ ] Fruits
- [ ] Wines
- [ ] Salt, sugar, honey, maple syrup
- [ ] Sours (e.g., lemon juice, lime juice, apple cider vinegar)

BOTANICAL PREPARATIONS

- [ ] Infused spirits
- [ ] Tinctures
- [ ] Bitters
- [ ] Glycerites
- [ ] Infusions/teas
- [ ] Syrups
- [ ] Vinegars

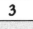

Foundational Preparations

When it comes to mixing, shaking, and stirring your way to botanical mixed drink success, there are some foundational preparations you'll want to know how to make—and possibly have on hand—to make creating your favorite drinks a bit easier.

We'll start by briefly explaining the purpose of each of these components and then share the steps you can take to make these foundational preparations yourself using the herbs of your choice.

HERB-INFUSED BASE SPIRITS

Infusing base spirits (various types of alcohol) with fragrant, flavorful herbs and foods is an easy way to give mixed drinks a botanical element.

Because the aromatic components of a plant are one of the first things to be extracted when making alcohol infusions, infusion times are much shorter than if you were making an herbal tincture, where you are trying to extract more than scent and flavor from the plant. Infusion times for base spirits can range from 3 hours to 14 days, depending on the botanical you are using and desired flavor. We've included a handy table with suggested infusion times for various botanicals that you can use as a guide when making your herb-infused base spirits.

INFUSION TIMES FOR BOTANICAL SPIRITS

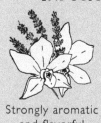 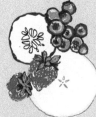 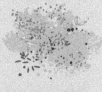

Strongly aromatic and flavorful botanicals, such as lavender flower bud and vanilla bean	Fresh herbs, citrus fruits, conifer needles, fresh roots	Fresh fruits and vegetables	Dried herbs and spices that lack a strong aroma or flavor
3-24 hours	1-3 days	3-7 days	Up to 14 days

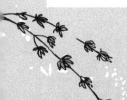

Now that you have a sense of how long to infuse botanical ingredients in alcohol, the next thing to consider is how much plant material to use.

You'll notice that the Basic Botanical Base Spirit recipe on the next page calls for a wide range where the botanical measurement is concerned (2 teaspoons to 3 tablespoons of fresh plant material and 1 teaspoon to 1½ tablespoons of dried plant material). As mentioned on the previous page, aromatic components differ from plant to plant. You may find that using a couple of teaspoons of one botanical (ginger, for example) is more than enough, while using a few tablespoons of another plant part, such as rose petals, doesn't quite give you enough of the flavor you're looking for. The amount of plant material you use will also vary depending on whether you are using fresh or dried plant material, the age of your plant material, and what type of alcohol you are using. For example, you may need to use more botanical material if you're infusing it into a flavorful alcohol, such as gin or rum, versus a more neutral alcohol, such as vodka.

See the table below for suggested amounts of plant material used for particular infused spirits called for in the recipes, although feel free to experiment to suit your taste preference!

On the following pages you will find several basic recipes for making some foundational herb-infused alcohols commonly found in mixed drink recipes. Remember that various herbs can be substituted in these recipes to fit the needs of the individual drink you are trying to create.

INFUSED SPIRITS

Herbs and spices that lack a strong aroma or flavor in a flavorful alcohol (e.g., dandelion flower, elderflower, violet, or calendula infused in gin or rum)	Herbs and spices that lack a strong aroma or flavor in a neutral alcohol (e.g., dandelion flower, elderflower, violet, or calendula infused in vodka)	Aromatic botanicals infused in a flavorful alcohol (e.g., lavender, rosemary, tulsi, or pine infused in gin or rum)	Aromatic botanicals infused in a neutral alcohol (e.g., lavender, rosemary, tulsi, or pine infused in vodka)	Fruits and vegetables
AMOUNT OF PLANT MATERIAL PER 1 CUP (8 FL OZ) ALCOHOL				
2–3 tbsp fresh plant material 1–1½ tbsp dried plant material	1–2 tbsp fresh plant material 2–3 tsp dried plant material	1–2 tbsp fresh plant material 2–3 tsp dried plant material	2–3 tsp fresh plant material 1–2 tsp dried plant material	¼–½ cup fresh fruit or vegetable ⅛–¼ cup dried fruit or vegetable

BASIC BOTANICAL BASE SPIRIT

Botanically infused base spirits serve as a foundation for most cocktail recipes. They are easy to make, can be used in various recipes to add color, flavor, and interest to a drink, and have a long shelf life of 1-2 years or more when stored in a cool, dark location. Feel free to double or triple the recipe if desired!

INGREDIENTS

2 tsp-3 tbsp fresh botanicals (1 tsp-1½ tbsp if using dried) or ¼-½ cup fresh fruit or vegetable (⅛-¼ cup if using dried)

8 fl oz (240 mL) alcohol of your choice (e.g., bourbon, brandy, gin, rum, scotch, or vodka)

DIRECTIONS

Combine the plant material and alcohol in a clean glass canning jar with a lid.

Place a piece of natural waxed paper between the jar and the lid, then seal. Label the jar, shake, and place in a dark location for 3 hours to 14 days, depending on the botanical you are using. Please refer to the Infusion Times for Botanical Spirits table for suggested infusion times.

When the desired infusion time has passed, open the jar and taste the alcohol. If the plant flavor is coming through, you can strain and bottle the infused spirit at this point. If you want the flavor to be more pronounced, leave it for another day before tasting again. You may also need to add additional herbs depending on the strength of the plant material and the flavor of the alcohol you are using. Continue tasting each day until you get the flavor you are after. Be careful not to infuse plants with bitter properties for too long, or the alcohol will develop a bitter flavor. If this happens, you can use it as a bitter in drink recipes that call for that taste component.

When you are satisfied with the flavor, strain the mixture through a fine-mesh sieve (lined with an unbleached coffee filter if needed to remove tiny herb particles), and compost the plant material, reserving the finished liquid in a labeled container. Store in a cool, dark location and use within 1-2 years.

WILD VERMOUTH

Vermouth is a classic martini ingredient that can be used in many other mixed drink recipes or enjoyed on its own as a post-dinner digestif to support digestion after a heavy meal. The botanical components of this drink are endless and are typically made with a mixture of aromatic, carminative, and bitter herbs. Familiarize yourself with the process of making vermouth using the following recipe, and don't hesitate to experiment with different herbs and flavors each time you make it! Vermouth has a shelf life of 1-2 months and should be stored in a cool, dark location.

INGREDIENTS
1 bottle (750 mL) 100-proof alcohol, such as vodka, gin, or grappa
1 bottle (750 mL) dry white wine
4 tsp (17 g) sugar (more for sweet vermouth)
Your choice of aromatic, carminative, and bitter herbs:
  Aromatic options: lavender, lemon balm, rose, tulsi
  Carminative options: peppermint, ginger, thyme, rosemary
  Bitter options: chamomile, dandelion root, hops, orange peel, mugwort

DIRECTIONS
The first step to making vermouth is to create individual tinctures of the herbs you have chosen. You can use as many botanicals in your vermouth as you wish, but including at least one herb from each category (aromatics, carminatives, and bitters) is vital. Because tinctures don't need to be precise for botanical mixed drinks, you can use the folk method to make these.

For each tincture, fill a small glass jar (4-8 fl oz) half full of the dried botanical you want to use, and then fill the jar with the alcohol of your choice. Ideally, you want to have at least 1 fl oz (30 mL) of the final tincture to use. Because you will use varying amounts of each tincture based on your taste preferences, it's a good idea to have at least five tinctures on hand, preferably more, to work with.

Place a piece of natural waxed paper between the jar and the lid, label, and store in a dark location for up to 2 weeks, shaking daily—and tasting the liquid daily starting on day four.

Strain the liquid from the herbs using a fine-mesh sieve (lined with an unbleached coffee filter if needed to remove tiny herb particles) when it has reached a pleasing but potent flavor.

Compost the herbs and transfer the finished tincture to a labeled glass bottle.

Next, combine the bottle of dry white wine with sugar in a saucepan. The amount of sugar you use is up to you. If you want to make dry vermouth, use no more than 4 teaspoons. If you're going to make sweet vermouth, add more until you achieve the sweet flavor you desire. Sugar helps balance the bitter botanicals and highlights the different flavors of the aromatic and carminative herbs. Bring this mixture to a boil, then reduce the heat and simmer for just a couple minutes. Allow the mixture to cool before moving to the final step. If using a sugar alternative such as honey, heat over low heat just until the honey is dissolved.

Last, make a botanical vermouth that suits your taste buds! Transfer the wine and sugar mixture to a clean bowl. Begin adding measured amounts of various tinctures, one at a time, keeping careful track of which and how much of each tincture you use. It's best to begin by adding your primary bitters and then working to balance the flavor with additional aromatic and carminative tinctures, tasting the combination after each botanical is added until you have a flavor that is pleasing to you. Remember, tincture flavors will vary in strength depending on the botanicals used. Start with small amounts, such as 5-10 mL, and slowly increase from there. Keep track of the final ratio of bitter, aromatic, and carminative tinctures you use in your blend so you can replicate the recipe in the future, scaling the volume based on the size batch you want to make. Alternatively, create a tincture blend in a separate container: once the blend is to your liking, add the blend to the wine and sugar mixture.

Transfer the final mixture into a clean, labeled storage bottle and set aside for 24 hours so the flavors can meld together. Store in a cool, dark location and use within 1-2 months for the best flavor.

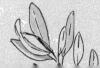

BASIC BOTANICAL LIQUEUR

Liqueurs are a type of sweetened alcohol with a syrupy consistency and are most often infused with botanicals to increase the flavor of a cocktail. While they are typically used in addition to base spirits, they can also be sipped on their own as a pre-dinner apéritif or post-dinner digestif. Liqueurs have a 6-12 month shelf life when stored in a cool, dark location. Feel free to double or triple the recipe if desired!

INGREDIENTS
1 cup fresh botanicals (½ cup if using dried) or ¼ pound fresh fruit (⅛ pound if using dried)
⅛ cup (25 g) sugar
8 fl oz (240 mL) alcohol of your choice (e.g., bourbon, brandy, gin, rum, scotch, vodka)
¼ fresh lemon, thinly sliced (optional – used to prevent flowers/fruits from oxidizing and turning brown)

DIRECTIONS
Combine all ingredients, except for lemon slices, in a glass canning jar with a lid.

Place the lemon slices on top to weigh the flowers/fruit down in the alcohol so they don't oxidize and turn brown. You can also use a small plate or weight of some sort if needed.

Place a piece of natural waxed paper between the jar and the lid, label, and store in a cool, dark location for 4 weeks. Once a week, remove the weight and/or lemons, stir the contents in the jar, and replace the weight/lemons before resealing the jar.

After 4 weeks, double strain the mixture through a fine-mesh sieve (lined with an unbleached coffee filter if needed to remove tiny herb particles). Compost the herbs, transfer the liqueur to a clean, labeled storage bottle, and store it in a cool, dark location. Use within 6-12 months.

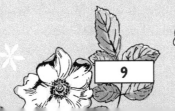

Alcohol Alternatives

If you prefer to skip the alcohol in your drinks and make a mocktail instead of a cocktail, you can substitute a botanical tea, glycerite, shrub, or syrup for the herb-infused spirit in the recipe.

Below are a couple of recipes that will walk you through the steps of creating basic botanical teas and glycerites to use in your botanical mixed drinks if you would like an alternative to alcohol. Shrubs and syrups are covered on page 15. Feel free to adapt these recipes to include various herbs of your choosing.

BASIC BOTANICAL TEA

Botanical teas, such as infusions, decoctions, or infusion-decoction combinations, can be a wonderful way to add color and flavor to your favorite mixed drinks. Not only that, but they are a great substitute for alcohol if you want to convert your cocktail into a mocktail! Infusions are typically made with soft herb parts, such as flowers and leaves, whereas decoctions are used for harder plant parts, such as roots, barks, and seeds. Infusions should be used within 24 hours of straining, decoctions should be used within 48 hours of straining, and both types of botanical tea should be stored in the refrigerator.

INGREDIENTS
2-6 tbsp fresh botanicals or 1-3 tbsp dried botanicals
8 fl oz (240 mL) water for infusions or 16 fl oz (480 mL) for decoctions

DIRECTIONS
To make a hot water infusion, bring water to a boil in a kettle or pot, then remove from heat. Place herbs in a heatproof mug or glass jar, pour hot water over the plant material and cover the container with a lid or plate to prevent volatile oils from escaping with the steam. Steep for 5-20 minutes (or 8 hours to overnight for a long-steeped infusion). Steeping time can vary depending on the herb and other factors, such as the desired flavor

and strength. When the desired steeping time has passed, strain the mixture through a fine-mesh sieve (lined with an unbleached coffee filter if needed to remove tiny herb particles), compost the herbs, and transfer the liquid to a clean container for use or storage. Refrigerate and use within 24 hours.

To make a cool water infusion, place herbs in a mug or glass jar, pour room temperature water over the plant material, and cover the container with a lid or plate. Steep on the counter or in the refrigerator for 4-8 hours, or overnight for a long-steeped infusion, depending on the herb and other factors, such as the desired flavor and strength. When the desired steeping time has passed, strain the mixture through a fine-mesh sieve (lined with an unbleached coffee filter if needed to remove tiny herb particles), compost the herbs, and transfer the liquid to a clean container for use or storage. Refrigerate and use within 24 hours.

To make a decoction, soak the herbs overnight to soften the plant material (optional) before placing them in a saucepan. Bring the herb and water mixture to a boil, then immediately reduce the heat to allow the mixture to simmer until the liquid has reduced by half to 8 fl oz (240 mL). Strain the mixture through a fine-mesh sieve (lined with an unbleached coffee filter if needed to remove tiny herb particles), compost the herbs, and transfer the liquid to a clean container for use or storage. Refrigerate and use within 48 hours.

To make an infusion-decoction combination, follow the steps for making a decoction above using only the hard herb parts called for in the recipe. Once the liquid in the saucepan has been reduced by half, remove from heat and then add the soft herb parts and steep, covered, for another 5-20 minutes to extract the desired flavor and potency from the herbs. When the desired steeping time has passed, strain the mixture through a fine-mesh sieve (lined with an unbleached coffee filter if needed to remove tiny herb particles), compost the herbs, and transfer the liquid to a clean container for use or storage. Refrigerate and use within 24 hours.

Basic Botanical Glycerite

Glycerites are a great way to add color, flavor, and sweetness to mixed drink recipes without impacting blood sugar levels. This herbal preparation is great for those looking to make their cocktail and mocktail recipes sugar- and alcohol-free. Glycerites have a shelf life of 1 year and should be stored in a cool, dark location.

INGREDIENTS
½ cup fresh botanicals or ¼ cup dried botanicals
Food-grade vegetable glycerin
Boiled water

DIRECTIONS
Place herbs into a clean glass canning jar with a lid.

If using dried herbs, add enough just-boiled water to wet the herb. (This step is unnecessary when using fresh herb(s) as they already contain water.) You want to be able to press the plant material with the back of a clean spoon and see a small amount of water squeeze out, but you don't want so much water that the plant material is floating in it. Cover the rehydrated herbs with glycerin, using just enough to cover the herbs by 1 inch.

If using fresh herbs, simply place them in a jar and fill it with glycerin, using just enough to cover the herbs by 1 inch.

Place a piece of natural waxed paper between the jar and the lid and seal. Label the jar, shake, and place it in a cool, dark location for 4–6 weeks, visiting every few days to give the jar a shake.

Strain the mixture through a fine-mesh sieve (lined with an unbleached coffee filter if needed to remove tiny herb particles), when time is up. It can be helpful to gently warm the jar in a water bath on the stove before straining to help thin the liquid so it passes through the sieve quickly.

Compost the herbs and transfer the glycerite to a clean, labeled storage bottle. Store in a cool, dark location. Glycerites that contain at least 55% glycerin typically have a shelf life of 1 year.

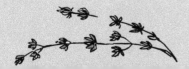

Botanical Salts, Sugars, Syrups, & Shrubs

You can easily elevate mixed drinks with botanical salts and sugars, both of which are used for rimming glasses, and syrups and shrubs, which add a sweet component to mixed drinks. Let's first discuss using botanical salts and sugars in mixed drinks before moving on to botanical syrups and shrubs.

BOTANICAL SALTS AND SUGARS

Salt comes in a variety of colors and flavors and can be blended with herbs to add a savory quality and cut the bitterness of a drink. You can also combine herbs with unbleached, non-GMO cane sugar (or maple, coconut, or date sugar as a sugar alternative) to add sweetness to a drink or garnish the glass's rim with some color.

To rim a glass, place 1 teaspoon of an herbal salt or sugar mix on a small plate. Next, rub a slice of citrus or a small amount of water, honey, maple syrup, or glycerite along the rim of a glass with your finger, and then turn the glass upside down and dip the moistened rim in the herbal salt or sugar mixture. Feel free to rim the entire glass or half of the glass, as desired.

On the following page, you will find a basic recipe for making your own botanical salts and sugars to use in mixed drink recipes. Remember that various herbs can be used in this recipe to fit the needs of the individual drink you are trying to create.

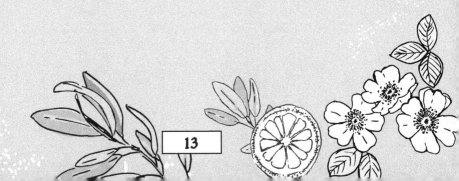

BOTANICAL SALTS AND SUGARS

Botanical salts and sugars are a lovely garnish for mixed drinks and really go a long way to boost the flavor (and wow factor!) of a drink. Feel free to rim the entire glass or only rim half if you're unsure whether or not the person drinking it will like a rimmed garnish. Botanical salts and sugars made with fresh herbs are shelf stable for 2 weeks and should be refrigerated. Those made with dried herbs are shelf stable for 2-3 months and can be stored in a cool, dark location.

INGREDIENTS
2 tsp fresh botanicals or 1 tsp dried botanicals
½-1 tsp (3-6 g) fine-grain salt
OR
½-1 tsp (2-4 g) unbleached, non-GMO cane sugar or sugar alternative

DIRECTIONS
If using fresh botanicals, chop finely using a knife.

If using dried botanicals, place in a mortar and pestle, coffee grinder, or small blender and gently break the herb apart into smaller pieces. When using a coffee grinder or blender, use quick short pulses as you don't want to powder the herb!

Next, combine the herb and salt or sugar in a small bowl and mix well.

When you're ready to rim the glass, transfer the botanical salt or sugar to a plate. Rub a small amount of water along the rim of a glass with your finger, and then dip the moistened rim in the herbal salt mixture. You can also moisten the rim of the glass with a citrus wedge, honey, maple syrup, or glycerite if you wish.

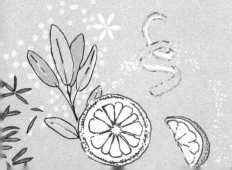

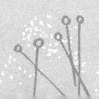

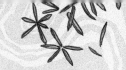

BOTANICAL SYRUPS AND SHRUBS

Syrups and shrubs are a common addition to mixed drink recipes that can be enhanced with botanicals and help bring balance to bitter or sour drinks. While unbleached, non-GMO cane sugar is most often used when making these types of mixed drink preparations, honey or other sugar alternatives can also be used.

On this and the following pages, you will find some basic recipes for making your own syrups and shrubs to use in your mixed drink recipes. Remember that various herbs can be substituted in these recipes to fit the needs of the individual drink you are trying to create.

BASIC SIMPLE SYRUP

Simple syrups are an easy way to balance a mixed drink with some sweet flavoring. Use a 1:1 ratio of sugar to water to make a simple syrup that has a subtle sweetness and will last 2-4 weeks in the refrigerator. For more sweetness and extended shelf life, use a 2:1 ratio of sugar to water to make a rich syrup that will last approximately 12 months when refrigerated.

INGREDIENTS
1-2 cups (200-400 g) non-GMO cane sugar or sugar alternative
1 cup (8 fl oz or 240 mL) water

DIRECTIONS
Combine sugar and water in a saucepan and heat over low heat, stirring until the sugar is completely dissolved.

Allow syrup to cool before bottling and labeling. Store syrup in the refrigerator and use within 2-4 weeks for a 1:1 syrup and 12 months for a 2:1 syrup.

BASIC BOTANICAL SYRUP

Botanical syrups are a perfect way to add color, flavor, and sweetness to your mixed drinks and bring some balance to overly strong, bitter, or sour drinks. Botanical syrups should be refrigerated, and have a 2-4 week shelf life if made with a 1:1 ratio of sugar to water and approximately 12 months if made with a 2:1 ratio of sugar to water.

INGREDIENTS
1-2 cups (200-400 g) unbleached, non-GMO cane sugar or sugar alternative
1 cup (8 fl oz or 240 mL) water
2-4 tbsp dried herb

DIRECTIONS
Combine sugar and water in a saucepan and heat over low heat, stirring until the sugar is completely dissolved.

Add the herb to the liquid. Less herb will result in a lighter color and milder flavor, whereas more herb will be more potent on both accounts. Stir to mix the botanicals into the liquid, and cover the saucepan with a lid to steep for 5 minutes. Taste to see if enough of the botanical flavor has transferred to the syrup. If not, cover with the lid and wait another 5 minutes before testing again.

Once you are satisfied with the syrup's flavor, strain the mixture through a fine-mesh sieve (lined with an unbleached coffee filter if needed to remove tiny herb particles).

Compost the herbs and allow the syrup to cool before bottling and labeling. Store syrup in the refrigerator and use within 2-4 weeks for a 1:1 syrup and 12 months for a 2:1 syrup.

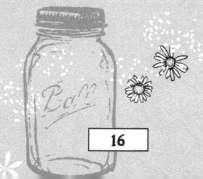

BASIC BOTANICAL SHRUB

Shrubs are a great way to add a hint of sweet and sour flavor to your mixed drinks. They are typically made with fruit, herbs, spices, and even vegetables, giving them a wide range of complex flavors. Shrubs can be made using both a hot or cold process method. They have a shelf life of 6 weeks and should be stored in the refrigerator.

INGREDIENTS
1 cup fresh plant material (fruit, vegetables, or botanicals), lightly crushed (½ cup if using spices or highly aromatic botanicals)
8 fl oz (240 mL) water (hot process method only)
1 cup unbleached, non-GMO cane sugar or sugar alternative
8 fl oz (240 mL) apple cider vinegar

DIRECTIONS
To make a cold process shrub, prepare 1 cup of fresh plant material by thoroughly washing it, then place it in a bowl and crush it to break the cell walls open. Add 1 cup of sugar and stir to combine the mixture thoroughly. Cover the bowl and place in the refrigerator for at least 4 hours, or up to 2 days. Before taking the bowl out of the refrigerator, check that the mixture has become very liquidy and juicy. Strain through a fine-mesh sieve (lined with an unbleached coffee filter if needed to remove tiny particles) and compost or reserve for another use. Transfer the liquid to a quart-sized glass canning jar, add 8 fl oz (240 mL) of vinegar, and stir to combine. Place a piece of natural waxed paper between the jar and lid, cap, and label the jar. Refrigerate for up to 6 weeks, shaking the shrub periodically to help blend and dissolve the sugar.

To make a hot process shrub, add 1 cup of sugar and 8 fl oz (240 mL) of water to a saucepan and heat over medium heat, stirring the mixture until the sugar dissolves completely. Next, prepare 1 cup of fresh plant material by thoroughly washing and placing it in the saucepan, crushing it to break the cell walls open, and stirring to combine it with the sugar and water mixture. Simmer for another 10-15 minutes until the plant material has thoroughly infused into the syrup. Allow the mixture to cool and then strain through a fine-mesh sieve to remove the chunks of plant material, which you can compost or reserve for another use. Transfer the liquid to a quart-sized glass canning jar, add 8 fl oz (240 mL) of vinegar, and stir to combine. Place a piece of natural waxed paper between the jar and lid, cap, and label the jar. Refrigerate for up to 6 weeks, shaking the shrub periodically to help blend and keep the sugar dissolved.

HERBAL BITTERS and TINCTURES

When making botanical mixed drinks, both herbal bitters and tinctures can be used to add important characteristics to your drink.

Bitterness is an essential component of a great mixed drink as it helps to balance out any strong, sweet, or acidic qualities of the other ingredients, and as an added bonus the bitter flavor helps to perk up digestion!

When making traditional herbal bitters for cocktails, you can either use a single bitter herb—called a simple—or a combination of herbs to make a bitter tincture using alcohol. While there is an entire art to formulating bitters for mixed drinks, in this recipe book we are keeping things straightforward by using simple bitters in our recipes but feel free to substitute with your favorite bitters blend, if desired.

You can also take bitter herbs and infuse them into vinegar to make what we call "vinegar bitters" to help bring a bit of that bitter balance to your botanical mocktails as well.

Tinctures, on the other hand, are often called for in mixed drink recipes for wellness-supporting purposes. Tinctures are made the same way as bitters, either as a simple or a blend of herbs.

In the recipes in this book, we use the term "bitters" if the herbal tincture is primarily bitter in flavor, and "tincture" if it has additional purposes other than use as a bitter.

On the following pages, you will find basic recipes for making both herbal bitters and herbal vinegar bitters. Remember that various herbs can be used in these recipes to fit the needs of the individual drink you are trying to create.

Basic Botanical Bitters and Tinctures

Bitters are easy to make and provide the perfect finishing touch to many mixed drink recipes. They are often referred to as the "salt and pepper" of a drink—only a dash or two is needed. Tinctures can add a variety of herbal actions to a drink and are typically added by the half teaspoon or teaspoon to mixed drinks. Bitters and tinctures have a shelf life of 1-2 years or more and should be stored in a cool, dry location.

INGREDIENTS
1 oz (28 g) fresh botanicals or ½ oz (14 g) dried botanicals: if making bitters, choose a bitter herb such as chamomile, dandelion root, hops, orange peel, mugwort, etc.
4 fl oz (120 mL) 40-50% (80-100 proof) alcohol, such as vodka or brandy

DIRECTIONS
Begin by weighing the plant material on a kitchen scale and placing it in a clean glass canning jar with a lid.

Next, measure out the alcohol in a glass measuring cup. Pour this over the herbs, then cover the jar with a piece of natural waxed paper and a lid. Label and store in a warm, dark location for 4-6 weeks, shaking daily if possible.

Strain the mixture through a fine-mesh sieve (lined with an unbleached coffee filter if needed to remove tiny herb particles) when time is up. Compost the herbs and transfer the reserved liquid to a dark-colored glass bottle with a dropper top and label. Store in a cool, dark location and use within 1-2 years.

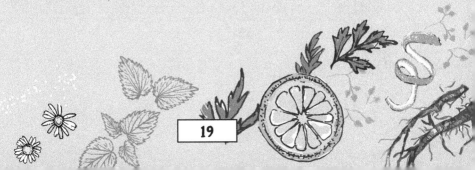

BASIC VINEGAR BITTERS AND TINCTURES

Vinegar is an excellent solvent for extracting the bitter properties of plant material, making it a suitable alternative to the classic alcohol-based bitters called for in mixed drink recipes. Additionally, it can be used as an alternative to alcohol when making a tincture. Because it also offers a sour component, you will want to keep this in mind when using it in drink recipes, perhaps decreasing or removing any acidic ingredients called for in the recipe. Vinegar bitters and tinctures have a shelf life of 6 months and should be stored in a cool, dark location.

INGREDIENTS
1 oz (28 g) fresh botanicals or ½ oz (14 g) dried botanicals; if making bitters, choose a bitter herb such as chamomile, dandelion root, hops, orange peel, mugwort, etc.
4 fl oz (120 mL) apple cider vinegar

DIRECTIONS
Begin by weighing the plant material on a kitchen scale and placing it in a clean glass canning jar with a lid.

Next, measure out the vinegar in a glass measuring cup. Pour this over the herbs, then cover the jar with a piece of natural waxed paper and a lid. Label and store in a warm, dark location for 4–6 weeks, shaking daily if possible.

Strain the mixture through a fine-mesh sieve (lined with an unbleached coffee filter if needed to remove tiny herb particles) when time is up. Compost the herbs and transfer the reserved liquid to a labeled dark-colored glass bottle with a dropper top and store in the refrigerator. If you use dried herbs, you do not have to refrigerate the vinegar. Use it within 6 months.

Troubleshooting
Herb-to-Liquid Ratios in Tinctures

Depending on the bitter herbs you use, you may find that there isn't enough alcohol or vinegar to cover the herbs. In this situation, you have a couple of options.

Your first option is to transfer the herb and alcohol or herb and vinegar mixture to a small blender and blend it to chop the plant material into smaller pieces. This will help to reduce the bulk of the plant material and expose more of its surface area, often allowing the alcohol or vinegar to cover the plant material and better extract its constituents. If the alcohol does not fully cover the plant material after blending the mixture together, it's a good idea to move on to the next option.

The second option is to increase the amount of alcohol or vinegar you use in your bitter tincture. To do this, measure out another 2 fl oz (60 mL) of alcohol or vinegar and add this to the jar. If that amount of alcohol or vinegar is enough to cover the plant material, move on to the remaining steps. If not, repeat this again with another 2 fl oz of alcohol or vinegar.

HERBAL SOURS

The last component of a mixed drink that we'll discuss here is an acidic one, which can come from vinegar, unripe or acidic fruits, sour berries, and even wine. Acids in drinks help to counter the sweetness of other ingredients, adding a level of satisfying savoriness that leaves you wanting another sip.

On the following page, you will find a basic recipe for a botanical vinegar. Remember that various herbs can be used in this recipe to fit the needs of the individual drink you are trying to create.

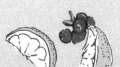

BASIC BOTANICAL VINEGAR

Botanical vinegars are so versatile. They are not only used as the sour component of a mixed drink recipe, but they can also be used in your meals, like in a healthy salad vinaigrette. Botanical vinegars made with fresh herbs have a shelf life of 6 months and should be refrigerated. Botanical vinegars made with dried herbs have a shelf life of 6 months when stored in a cool, dark location or longer if refrigerated.

INGREDIENTS
Fresh or dried botanicals
Apple cider vinegar

DIRECTIONS
Begin by filling a glass jar with fresh herbs, packing the jar ¾ full. If using dried herbs, you will only fill your jar ⅓ of the way full.

Next, fill the jar with enough vinegar to cover the herbs by 1 inch.

Cover the jar with a piece of natural waxed paper and a lid. Label and store in a warm, dark location for 1 week, shaking daily if possible. After 1 week, open the jar and taste the vinegar. If you enjoy the flavor, you can decant the mixture now. If you want the flavor to be stronger, let the mixture sit for several more days before tasting again.

When you are happy with the flavor, strain the mixture through a fine-mesh sieve (lined with an unbleached coffee filter if needed to remove tiny herb particles), and compost the herbs. Transfer the reserved liquid to a labeled storage container and store it in the refrigerator. If you use dried herbs, you do not have to refrigerate the vinegar. Use it within 6 months.

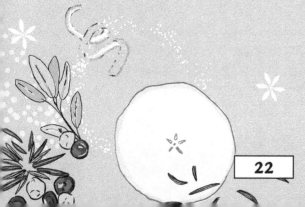

CHAPTER TWO

BOTANICAL MIXED DRINKS RESOURCES

Whether you are whipping up a pre-dinner apéritif or serving drinks to guests at a holiday party, we've gathered some creative and tasty botanical mixed drink recipes together in one place to help you do that very thing. We hope you enjoy these as much as we do and find yourself coming back to these recipes again and again!

NOTES

Here are some important notes to keep in mind as you peruse and utilize the recipes:

Recipes yield 1 drink unless otherwise noted.

All ingredients are dried unless otherwise noted. We recommend choosing organic, sustainably grown ingredients, if possible.

Refer to the Foundational Preparations on pages 4-22 of Chapter 1 to learn how to make basic herb-infused botanical spirits, liqueurs, teas, glycerites, syrups, shrubs, salts and sugars, bitters, and vinegars, as well as each preparation's shelf-life recommendations.

Before making a recipe, it's a good idea to review the ingredients so that you can prepare any infused spirits, syrups, vinegars, bitters, teas, etc. ahead of time. Some of these ingredients need to infuse for several weeks, and you'll want to make sure you have everything on hand the day you plan to make your botanical mixed drink(s)! To help you in doing that, we have compiled a list of herb-infused preparations that appear in multiple recipes in the **Botanical Staple Preparations Table** on page 25 so you can start to create your own mixed drinks pantry! However, there are many additional single-use ingredients, such as herbal bitters and syrups, that you may also want to prepare in advance.

Plant parts used in recipes are indicated in the **Plant Names & Parts Table** on page 28; if multiple plant parts are listed for a particular plant, the part used in a particular recipe is noted directly in the recipe ingredient list.

While recipes that include herbal bitters are formulated with a particular bitter plant in mind, feel free to substitute a different bitter if you prefer.

All conversions from milliliter (mL) to fluid ounce (fl oz) are rounded to the nearest ten (assuming 30 mL/fl oz) to be user friendly. We recommend using an online conversion calculator if you want an exact conversion.

MEASUREMENT CONVERSIONS

1 fl oz	2 tbsp	6 tsp	30 mL

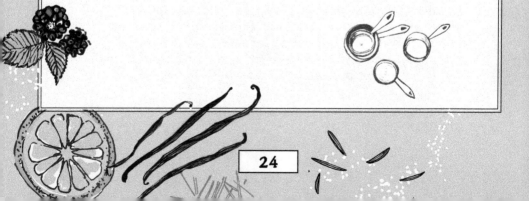

BOTANICAL STAPLE PREPARATIONS

ANISE HYSSOP SYRUP	Blue *Althaea* Delight Brandy *Agastache* Evergreen Highball
CHAMOMILE BITTERS OR TINCTURE	Blue *Althaea* Delight Kerchief and Cap Hot Brandy NightCap Tonic Perch on Bedford Common Cocktail Thyme to Sleep
CHERRY SHRUB	Cheery Cherry Spritzer Kerchief and Cap Hot Brandy
DANDELION FLOWER SYRUP	Cleavers Ginger Melon Agua Fresca Spring Dandy Whiskey Sour
ELDERBERRY SYRUP	Rum to Bed Sweet Spiced Wine
ELDERFLOWER LIQUEUR (OR ELDERFLOWER GLYCERITE)	Chamomile and Elderflower Iced Toddy Flora Forager Collins Purple Blossom
GINGER SYRUP	Blue Ginger Fizz Fruity Fizz High-C Toddy Pineapple Ginger Frozen Daiquiri Red Mule Smoke and Mirrors Spring Sting
GINGER VODKA	Cleavers Ginger Melon Agua Fresca Pear and Ginger Blitz
HAWTHORN BERRY SYRUP	Bright and Cheery Heart's Ease Gin and Tonic
HIBISCUS VODKA	Blue Ginger Fizz Hibiscus Lemon Drop
HOPS TINCTURE	NightCap Tonic Rum to Bed Thyme to Sleep
LAVENDER GIN	Cucumber Lavender-Ade Flora Forager Collins Southwest Sundowner

LEMON BALM SYRUP	Calming Watermelon Spritzer Garden Mint Old Fashioned
MINT BOURBON	Garden Mint Old Fashioned Kentucky Mint Refresher
MUGWORT SCOTCH	Minty Rose Mojito Mugwort Fig Smash Smoke and Mirrors
ORANGE BITTERS (OR ORANGE VINEGAR)	Bloody Rosemary Flora Forager Collins Orange Blossom Apéritif Rosemary Citrus Old Fashioned Violet Fizz
ORANGE LIQUEUR	Bloody Rosemary Mugwort Fig Smash Perch on Bedford Common Cocktail
ORANGE SYRUP	Bloody Rosemary Midwinter Digestif Shrub Mugwort Fig Smash Rosemary Citrus Old Fashioned
PASSIONFLOWER TINCTURE	Fruity Fizz NightCap Tonic Thyme to Sleep
PINE GIN	Pepper and Pine Woodland Gimlet
ROSE PETAL GIN	Heart's Ease Gin and Tonic Lover's Secret Elixir
ROSE PETAL SUGAR	Cardamom Rose Eggnog Pineapple Ginger Frozen Daiquiri Really Rosy Faux Rosé Rosy Tulsi-Tini
ROSE PETAL SYRUP	Flora Forager Collins Holiday Hot Cacao Minty Rose Mojito Really Rosy Faux Rosé Rosy Tulsi-Tini
ROSE PETAL VODKA	Brandy *Agastache* Cardamom Rose Eggnog

ROSEHIP SYRUP	Hibiscus Lemon Drop High-C Toddy Rosehip Cranberry Margarita Sumac 75 Sweet Spiced Wine
ROSEMARY RUM	Rosemary Rhubarb Rosemary Roger
ROSEMARY SYRUP	Bloody Rosemary Gin Wiz Rosemary Rhubarb Woodland Gimlet
SKULLCAP TINCTURE	Brandy *Agastache* Fruity Fizz Garden Mint Old Fashioned
TULSI SYRUP	Lung Love Cordial Tulsi Lime Margarita
TULSI VODKA	Rosy Tulsi-Tini Tulsi Blossom Spritzer
VANILLA EXTRACT	Chai-Spiced Apple Cider Lover's Secret Elixir Spring Clean Chai Warm and Welcome Liqueur
VANILLA SYRUP	Cheery Cherry Spritzer Perch on Bedford Common Cocktail Rosemary Roger
VIOLET SYRUP	Purple Blossom Violet Fizz
WILD VERMOUTH	Perch on Bedford Common Cocktail Rosy Tulsi-Tini

Plant Names & Parts

COMMON NAME	BINOMIAL	PLANT PART USED in RECIPES
ALLSPICE	*Pimenta dioica*	Berry
ANGELICA	*Angelica archangelica*	Root
ANISE	*Pimpinella anisum*	Seed
ANISE HYSSOP	*Agastache foeniculum*	Aerial parts
ASHWAGANDHA	*Withania somnifera*	Root
ASTRAGALUS	*Astragalus mongholicus*	Root
BASIL	*Ocimum basilicum*	Leaf
BURDOCK	*Arctium lappa*	Root
CACAO	*Theobroma cacao*	Fruit
CALENDULA	*Calendula officinalis*	Flower
CALIFORNIA POPPY	*Escholschzia californica*	Whole plant
CARDAMOM	*Elettaria cardamomum*	Pod and seed
CATNIP	*Nepeta cataria*	Aerial parts
CAYENNE	*Capsicum annuum*	Fruit
CHAMOMILE	*Matricaria chamomilla*	Flower
CINNAMON	*Cinnamomum* spp.	Bark
CLEAVERS	*Galium aparine*	Aboveground parts
CLOVE	*Syzygium aromaticum*	Bud
COFFEE	*Coffea* spp.	Fruit
CORDYCEPS	*Cordyceps militaris*	Mushroom
DAMIANA	*Turnera diffusa*	Aerial parts
DANDELION	*Taraxacum officinale*	Flower and root
ELDER	*Sambucus nigra. S. canadensis*	Flower and berry
ELEUTHERO	*Eleutherococcus senticosus*	Root

FENNEL	*Foeniculum vulgare*	Seed
GINGER	*Zingiber officinale*	Rhizome
GINKGO	*Ginkgo biloba*	Leaf
GINSENG	*Panax* spp.	Root
GOLDENROD	*Solidago* spp.	Aerial parts
GOTU KOLA	*Centella asiatica*	Leaf
HAWTHORN	*Crataegus* spp.	Berry
HIBISCUS	*Hibiscus sabdariffa*	Calyx
HOPS	*Humulus lupulus*	Strobile
JUNIPER	*Juniperus communis*	Berry
LAVENDER	*Lavandula* spp.	Flower bud
LEMON	*Citrus* x *limon*	Peel
LEMON BALM	*Melissa officinalis*	Aerial parts
LICORICE	*Glycyrrhiza glabra*	Root
LILAC	*Syringa vulgaris*	Flower
LINDEN	*Tilia* spp.	Flower and bract
MAITAKE	*Grifola frondosa*	Mushroom
MARSHMALLOW	*Althaea officinalis*	Flower and root
MIMOSA	*Albizia julibrissin*	Flower
MOTHERWORT	*Leonurus cardiaca*	Aerial parts
MUGWORT	*Artemisia vulgaris*	Leaf
MULLEIN	*Verbascum thapsus*	Leaf
NETTLE	*Urtica dioica*	Leaf
NUTMEG	*Myristica fragrans*	Seed
OAT	*Avena sativa*	Milky tops
ORANGE	*Citrus* spp.	Peel

PASSIONFLOWER	*Passiflora incarnata*	Aerial parts
PEPPER	*Piper nigrum*	Fruit
PEPPERMINT	*Mentha x piperita*	Leaf
PINE	*Pinus* spp.	Needle
PINEAPPLE WEED	*Matricaria discoidea*	Flower
RED ROOIBOS	*Aspalathus linearis*	Leaf
REISHI	*Ganoderma* spp.	Mushroom
ROSE	*Rosa* spp.	Petal and hip
ROSEMARY	*Salvia rosmarinus*	Leaf
SAGE	*Salvia officinalis*	Leaf
SKULLCAP	*Scutellaria lateriflora*	Aerial parts
SPEARMINT	*Mentha spicata*	Leaf
SPRUCE	*Picea* spp.	Young needles (tips)
STAR ANISE	*Illicium verum*	Seed pod
SUMAC	*Rhus* spp.	Berry
TEA (black, green, white)	*Camellia sinensis*	Leaf
THYME	*Thymus vulgaris*	Leaf
TULSI	*Ocimum tenuiflorum*	Aerial parts
VALERIAN	*Valeriana officinalis*	Root
VANILLA	*Vanilla planifolia*	Pod
VIOLET	*Viola odorata. V. sororia*	Flower
WILD CHERRY	*Prunus serotina*	Bark
WOOD BETONY	*Betonica officinalis*	Aerial parts

Aerial parts refers to leaves and flowers.
Aboveground parts refers to stem, leaves, and flowers.

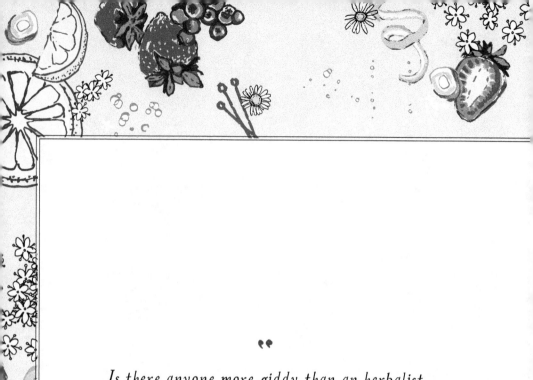

＂＂

Is there anyone more giddy than an herbalist in springtime? After a long winter, those first green shoots of nettle and dandelion are a glorious sight to behold.

HERBAL ACADEMY'S INTRODUCTORY HERBAL COURSE

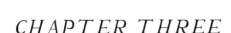

CHAPTER THREE

SPRING BOTANICAL MIXED DRINKS

Spring brings an abundance of fresh herbs and flowers emerging after months of dormancy. In celebration of this season of growth and renewal, these mixed drink recipes feature the finest spring botanicals, including cleavers, dandelion, nettle, violet, rose, and elderflower, and produce such as rhubarb and strawberries.

If you enjoy foraging, then we hope you'll grab your plant identification book and head outdoors to wildcraft your own fresh ingredients under the spring sun. Maybe you'll find the sweet blossoms of honeysuckle or stumble upon a lush patch of nettle. Whether you forage the ingredients or purchase them, the following drinks will share the taste of spring—imbued with a bubbly, floral freshness that preludes warm days to come.

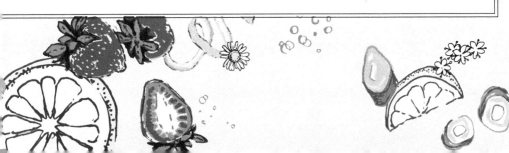

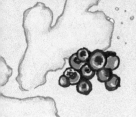

Blue Ginger
FIZZ

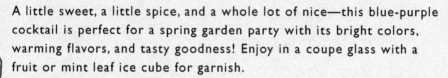

A little sweet, a little spice, and a whole lot of nice—this blue-purple cocktail is perfect for a spring garden party with its bright colors, warming flavors, and tasty goodness! Enjoy in a coupe glass with a fruit or mint leaf ice cube for garnish.

Yield: 30 fl oz, or 5 servings (6 fl oz each)

INGREDIENTS

15 fl oz (450 mL) carbonated water (or ginger beer), chilled

8 fl oz (240 mL) hibiscus vodka

4 fl oz (120 mL) ginger syrup (use simple syrup if using ginger beer)

2 cups fresh blueberries (extra for ice cube garnish, optional)

1 fresh lemon, sliced (extra for ice cube garnish, optional)

20 fresh mint leaves (extra for ice cube garnish, optional)

DIRECTIONS

To make ice cubes, fill an ice cube tray with extra blueberries, lemon peel slices, and/or chopped mint. Cover with water and freeze overnight.

In a bowl, mash 1 cup of blueberries and half of the mint leaves with hibiscus vodka and ginger syrup. Strain the mixture through a fine-mesh sieve and transfer the fruity liquid to a glass pitcher. Add the remaining whole blueberries, mint leaves, and lemon slices and chill in the refrigerator until ready to serve.

When ready to serve, add chilled carbonated water or ginger beer to the fruity liquid, gently stir to combine, and pour into coupe glasses.

Garnish by adding 2-3 ice cubes to each glass.

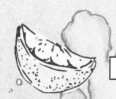

CHAMOMILE & ELDERFLOWER
Iced Toddy

The apple-like, floral nature of chamomile flowers blend beautifully with the oak undertones of aged whiskey. This surprisingly lovely combination is further enhanced with elderflower liqueur, a whimsical addition to any herbalist's bar. Add a drizzle of honey, and you're drinking a delightfully herbal, iced version of a classic hot toddy. Enjoy this cocktail in a rocks glass with extra chamomile or elder flowers or a lemon wheel for garnish.

INGREDIENTS

6 fl oz (180 mL) cooled chamomile tea
(or pineapple weed tea if available)

1½ fl oz (45 mL) whiskey

1 tsp (5 mL) honey (or other sweetener)

½ fl oz (15 mL) elderflower liqueur

Fresh chamomile flower, elderflower, or lemon wheel
for garnish (optional)

DIRECTIONS

Combine all ingredients, except garnish, in a glass canning jar.

Fill the jar ⅔ full of ice, cap, and shake hard for 20 seconds. Strain the liquid off the ice and pour it into a rocks glass.

Garnish with fresh chamomile flowers, elderflowers, or a floating lemon wheel (optional).

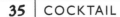

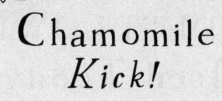

Chamomile
Kick!

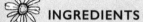

This refreshing cocktail is a healthier (but just as delicious) herbal twist on the classic moscow mule. Just like spring itself, it has elements that are warming and invigorating with a soothing, hopeful aftertaste. Enjoy over ice in a copper mug or rocks glass.

INGREDIENTS

2 fl oz (60 mL) cooled chamomile tea

2 fl oz (60 mL) vodka

½ fl oz (15 mL) chamomile syrup

1 fl oz (30 mL) freshly squeezed lime juice

½ tsp fresh ginger, minced

DIRECTIONS

Fill a copper mug or rocks glass with ice and set aside.

Combine all ingredients in a glass canning jar.

Fill the jar ⅔ full of ice, cap, and shake hard for 20 seconds. Strain the liquid off the ice and pour it over the ice into the copper mug or rocks glass.

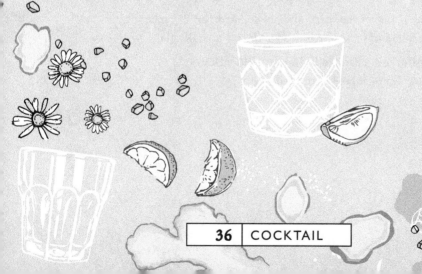

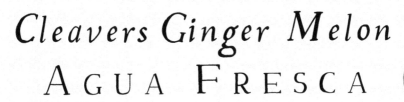

Cleavers Ginger Melon
AGUA FRESCA

Light and refreshing, this agua fresca can be enjoyed as a cocktail or a mocktail, depending on your preference. Traditionally served in group settings alongside light finger foods, this botanical version supports the body's detox functions and is a perfect fit for the spring season. Enjoy in stemless wine glasses with fresh mint leaves for garnish.

Yield: 56 fl oz, or 9 servings (6 fl oz each)

INGREDIENTS

32 fl oz (960 mL) water

1 cup fresh cleavers

1 cup fresh honeydew melon, chopped (or green grapes)

8 fl oz (240 mL) ginger vodka (or cooled ginger tea)

5 fl oz (150 mL) dandelion flower syrup

8 fl oz (240 mL) freshly squeezed lime juice

10 fresh mint leaves

Additional mint leaves for garnish (optional)

DIRECTIONS

Combine all ingredients, except additional mint leaves for garnish, in a blender and blend. Strain through a fine-mesh sieve to remove pulp. Compost the pulp and chill the remaining liquid in the refrigerator until time to serve.

When ready to serve, carefully pour mixture into stemless wine glasses.

Garnish with fresh mint leaves.

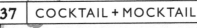

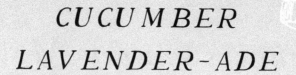

CUCUMBER LAVENDER-ADE

Late spring calls for the refreshing flavors of cucumber, lavender, and lemon all swirled together in this relaxing, colorful cocktail or mocktail that is sure to please you and your guests! Enjoy in a collins glass over ice with one or two lemon wheels as garnish.

INGREDIENTS

6 fl oz (180 mL) lemonade

2 fl oz (60 mL) lavender gin (or cooled lavender tea)

1 fresh cucumber, sliced

1-2 fresh lemon wheels for garnish (optional)

DIRECTIONS

To make a cocktail, combine the lemonade, lavender gin, and sliced cucumber in a glass canning jar.

To make a mocktail, combine the lemonade, lavender tea, and sliced cucumber in a glass canning jar.

Transfer mixture to the refrigerator to chill for 2-3 hours so flavors can combine.

When ready to serve, fill a collins glass with ice and wedge one or two lemon wheels between the glass and the ice, if desired. Strain the refrigerated mixture through a fine-mesh sieve to remove the cucumber slices, pour mixture into glass, and serve!

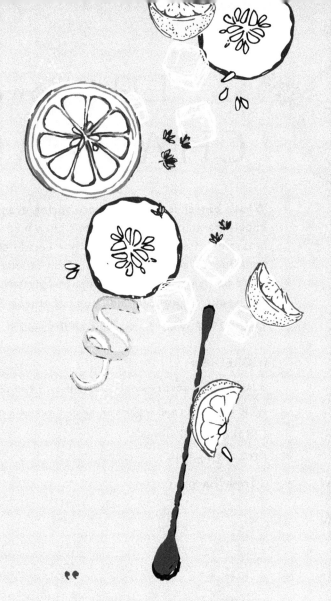

Spring is a reunion of sorts for herbalists—a time when we happily greet old friends as they once again emerge from the earth. The plants return from the underworld with their abundant gifts in tow, and we reestablish our connection with the earth through their beauty and nourishment.

THE HERBARIUM

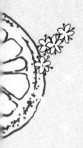

Elderflower
CHAMPAGNE

What's better for a festive late spring event than a nice glass of bubbly, particularly one that has been made from the creamy white blossoms of elderflower? This homemade champagne will tickle your guests' tongues and have them talking of this tasty treat for years to come! Enjoy in champagne glasses. Note: this recipe takes 1-2 weeks to prepare and requires sturdy flip-top glass bottles.

Yield: 129 fl oz, or 21 servings (6 fl oz each)

INGREDIENTS

8 large heads fresh elderflower (or ½–1 cup dried)

1½ lb (680 g) cane sugar (or sugar alternative)

128 fl oz (3.8 L) water

1 fl oz (30 mL) white wine vinegar

2 fresh lemons

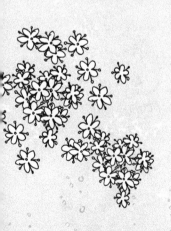

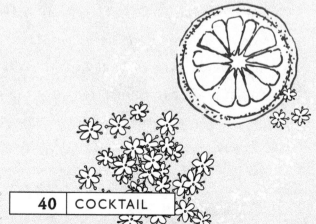

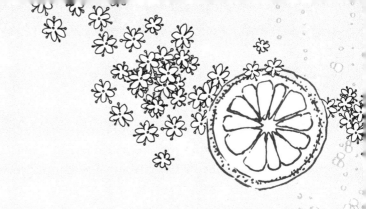

DIRECTIONS

Zest and juice two lemons. Combine lemon zest, juice, and peels along with other ingredients in a clean bucket or crock, and stir until sugar is dissolved and all components are thoroughly combined.

Cover the container with layered cheesecloth or a clean cotton towel to keep insects from getting into the liquid, and secure it with a string.

Place the container in a cool, dark location where it will not be disturbed for 24 hours.

After 24 hours, strain the mixture through a fine-mesh sieve to remove the elderflowers and lemons. Compost the elderflowers and lemons and transfer the liquid to glass flip-top bottles for storage.

Place the bottles in a cool, dark location and let ferment for 1 to 2 weeks. Carefully open the bottles daily to let the built-up gases from the fermentation process escape. This is called "burping," which will prevent the bottles from bursting under pressure. Transfer the bottles to the refrigerator for storage as soon as you have enough fizz present when you burp the bottles. Continue to burp the bottles every day or two to release the pressure.

When ready to serve, carefully pour into champagne glasses.

Flora Forager Collins

This ode to foraged late spring florals can be made as a mocktail or a cocktail and is a perfect botanical mixed drink for garden parties. It is light, fragrant, and refreshing. Enjoy in a collins glass over ice and garnish with fresh flowers, sprigs of culinary herbs, sweet berries, and a citrus twist.

INGREDIENTS

2 fl oz (60 mL) lavender gin (or cooled lavender tea)

½ fl oz (15 mL) elderflower liqueur (or elderflower glycerite)

½ fl oz (15 mL) rose petal syrup

¼ fl oz (7 mL) freshly squeezed lemon juice

1 dash (10 drops) orange bitters (or orange vinegar)

Carbonated water to taste

Fresh edible flowers, sprigs of culinary herbs, and/or sweet berries for garnish

10 drops hibiscus syrup (optional)

Fresh citrus twist for garnish (optional)

DIRECTIONS

Fill a collins glass with ice. Tuck fresh edible flowers, berries, and/or herb sprigs between the ice and the glass, and set it aside.

To make a cocktail, combine the lavender gin, elderflower liqueur, rose petal syrup, lemon juice, and orange bitters in a glass canning jar.

To make a mocktail, combine the lavender tea, elderflower glycerite, rose petal syrup, lemon juice, and orange vinegar in a glass canning jar.

Fill the jar ⅔ full of ice, cap, and shake hard for 20 seconds. Strain the liquid off the ice and pour it into the collins glass.

Add a citrus twist on top of the ice and any remaining berries or edible flowers you want to float on top of the drink, if desired.

Slowly pour carbonated water over the ice.

Using a pipette, place a small amount of hibiscus syrup in the bottom of the glass to give it a bold red coloring at the bottom, if desired.

Fruity Tooty
BRUNCH PUNCH

Brunch deserves to include a fun botanical drink of its own, and this version of brunch punch is just the thing for spring! This makes a large batch of punch, so invite plenty of friends and family over and enjoy in coupe glasses with chamomile sugar rims.

Yield: 125 fl oz, or 20 servings (6 fl oz each)

INGREDIENTS

68 fl oz (2 L) carbonated water

1 bottle (750 mL) champagne

16 fl oz (480 mL) orange juice

8 fl oz (240 mL) cranberry juice

8 fl oz (240 mL) chamomile liqueur (or chamomile glycerite)

1 cup fresh strawberries, sliced

½ cup fresh raspberries, whole

½ cup fresh blueberries, whole

Chamomile sugar for rimming (optional)

DIRECTIONS

Chill all ingredients in the refrigerator until ready to make the punch.

Rim coupe glasses with chamomile sugar to add an extra hint of sweetness to the drinks, if desired, and set it aside.

When ready to serve, combine all ingredients in a punch bowl and gently stir to combine. Ladle punch into coupe glasses, being careful not to disturb the chamomile sugar rim.

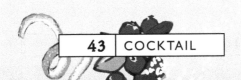

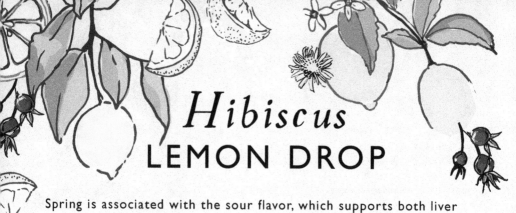

Hibiscus
LEMON DROP

Spring is associated with the sour flavor, which supports both liver and gut function, so what better way to embrace the benefits of this taste than with a botanical lemon drop cocktail? Enjoy as a cocktail or mocktail in a martini glass garnished with a lemon zest sugar rim.

INGREDIENTS

2 fl oz (60 mL) hibiscus vodka (or cooled hibiscus tea)

1 fl oz (30 mL) rosehip syrup

1 fl oz (30 mL) fresh squeezed lemon juice

1 dash (10 drops) dandelion root bitters (or dandelion root vinegar)

Lemon zest sugar for rimming (optional)

Fresh lemon slice for garnish (optional)

DIRECTIONS

Rim a martini glass with lemon zest sugar, if desired, and set it aside.

To make a cocktail, combine the hibiscus vodka, rosehip syrup, and lemon juice in a glass canning jar.

To make a mocktail, combine the hibiscus tea, rosehip syrup, and lemon juice in a glass canning jar.

Fill the jar ⅔ full of ice, cap, and shake hard for 20 seconds. Strain the liquid off the ice and pour into the martini glass, being careful not to disturb the sugar rim. Top with dandelion root bitters (for a cocktail) or dandelion root vinegar (for a mocktail).

Garnish with a lemon slice on the edge of the glass, if desired, and serve.

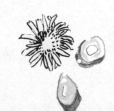

LAVENDER
CITRUS RUM PUNCH

Hosting a spring event or celebration for a group? If so, this tasty citrus punch cocktail will be quite the hit with guests, especially when they see the floral ice ring floating in the center! Serve in a punch bowl and enjoy in punch glasses.

Yield: 72 fl oz, or 12 servings (6 fl oz each)

INGREDIENTS

20 fl oz (600 mL) light rum

14 fl oz (420 mL) orange juice

14 fl oz (420 mL) grapefruit juice

12 fl oz (360 mL) lavender syrup

12 fl oz (360 mL) freshly squeezed lemon juice

Floral ice ring for garnish (optional)

DIRECTIONS

The day before your event, you will want to make a floral ice ring. To do this, fill a bundt pan ¼ full of water and place as many fresh edible flowers in it as you'd like—the more, the better. Place in the freezer; when frozen, the flowers will be at the top of the ice ring. Once frozen, fill the remainder of the pan with water and freeze again.

Also place ingredients in the refrigerator to chill the day before your event.

To make the punch, combine all the ingredients together and stir well. Taste test for sweetness and lavender flavor and adjust by adding more lavender syrup (or rum) to the mixture until you have it just right.

When you're ready to serve, pour the mixture into a punch bowl. To remove the floral ice ring from the bundt pan, place the pan in a bowl of warm water until the ice ring releases. Place the ice ring in the punch bowl, flower side up, which will keep your punch cool.

Ladle into punch glasses.

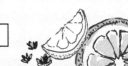

Minty Green
SANGRIA

Spring offers the return of many plants that nourish and support the body's cleansing pathways—helping to wake the body up from winter's slumber. As the first warm days of spring arrive, this minty green sangria is a perfect way to celebrate the warmth and light of the season with friends and family, and to welcome wellness into your year! Enjoy this cocktail in wine glasses.

Yield: 60 fl oz, or 10 servings (6 fl oz each)

INGREDIENTS

1 bottle (750 mL) white wine

32 fl oz (960 mL) water

2 tbsp green tea leaf

4 tbsp fresh cleavers

⅓ cup honey (or other sweetener)

2 fresh lemons, sliced

20 fresh peppermint leaves

DIRECTIONS

Bring water to a boil. As you wait for the water to boil, combine green tea leaf and fresh cleavers in a quart-sized heat-safe glass canning jar.

Pour boiled water over the plant material and steep for no more than 5 minutes to avoid the green tea becoming too bitter. Strain the mixture through a fine-mesh sieve, compost the plant material, and add the liquid to a serving pitcher. Allow to cool slightly. Add honey and stir until honey is dissolved, then allow to cool to room temperature.

When cool, add wine, lemon slices, and fresh peppermint leaves and immediately place in the refrigerator for 2-4 hours to chill before serving in wine glasses.

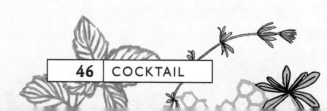

PERFECT
mint mojito

As a cold-hardy perennial, mint is always one of the first herbs that bounces back to life in early spring. The leaves are the star ingredient in mojitos, a classic Cuban cocktail made with white rum, fresh mint, lime juice, sparkling water, and sugar. Feel free to use a sugar alternative, such as honey or maple syrup, for a healthier twist. When making this mojito, it's best if you muddle the mint leaves directly in the glass you'll be serving it in (rather than in the glass jar). It's a small detail, but it makes a big difference! Enjoy in a collins glass over ice and garnish with fresh mint leaves.

INGREDIENTS

10 fresh mint leaves

½ lime, quartered

1½ fl oz (45 mL) white rum

¾ fl oz (20 mL) honey (or other sweetener)

¾ fl oz (20 mL) water

1½ fl oz (45 mL) carbonated water

Fresh mint leaves for garnish (optional)

DIRECTIONS

Add 10 mint leaves to the bottom of a collins glass, pressing the leaves against the sides of the glass with the back of a spoon to muddle them, releasing their aromatics into the glass.

Add 1 lime quarter to the glass and press down with a spoon to release the juice.

Fill the glass with crushed ice and set it aside.

Combine rum, honey, and water in a glass canning jar.

Fill the jar ⅔ full of ice, cap, and shake hard for 20 seconds. Strain the liquid off the ice and pour it into the collins glass. Top the glass with carbonated water and stir to combine.

Garnish with any extra fresh mint leaves, if desired.

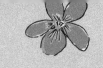

Purple *Blossom*

Based on the stormy morning cocktail with some extra violet
and elderflower love, this purple cocktail is the perfect way to
soak up the soothing sweetness of violets and the diaphanous joy
that elderflowers bring. Enjoy in a collins glass with fresh violet
flowers as a garnish.

INGREDIENTS

4 fl oz (120 mL) elderflower champagne, chilled (see recipe on page 40)
(or store-bought champagne)

1½ fl oz (45 mL) elderflower liqueur

1½ fl oz (45 mL) violet syrup

1 fl oz (30 mL) violet vinegar

Fresh violet flowers for garnish (optional)

DIRECTIONS

Fill a collins glass with ice and set aside.

Combine elderflower liqueur, violet syrup, and violet vinegar in a glass
canning jar.

Fill the jar ⅔ full of ice, cap, and shake hard for 20 seconds. Strain
the liquid off the ice and pour it into the collins glass. Top with chilled
elderflower champagne (or store-bought champagne), and stir to combine.

Garnish with fresh violet flowers, if desired.

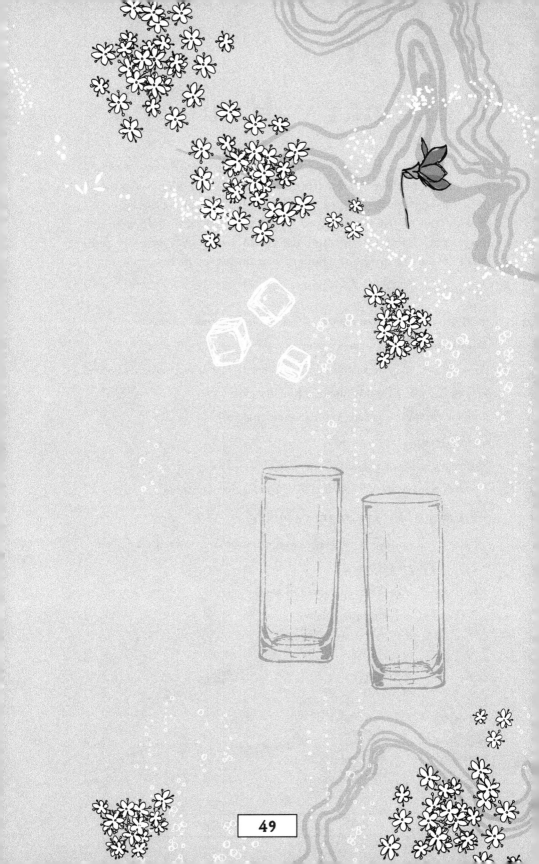

Rosemary Rhubarb

Where bitter meets sweet—let us introduce you to the rosemary rhubarb—a perfect combination of sweet, savory, and a wee bit of bitter thrown in for good measure. This refreshing cocktail or mocktail is just the thing to jump-start digestion before an *al fresco* meal. Enjoy in a martini glass with a rosemary salt rim and a fresh rosemary sprig and rhubarb ribbon for garnish.

INGREDIENTS

1½ fl oz (45 mL) rosemary rum (or cooled rosemary tea)

2 fl oz (60 mL) rosemary syrup

1½ fl oz (45 mL) Rhubarb and Strawberry Purée (ingredients below)

½ fl oz (15 mL) freshly squeezed lemon juice

5 drops cayenne tincture (or cayenne vinegar) (optional)

Carbonated water to taste

Rosemary salt for rimming (optional)

Fresh rosemary and rhubarb ribbon for garnish (optional)

RHUBARB AND STRAWBERRY PURÉE:

1 cup (3–4 stalks) fresh rhubarb, diced and steamed until softened

1 cup fresh strawberries

½ fl oz (15 mL) freshly squeezed lemon juice

2 fl oz (60 mL) simple syrup

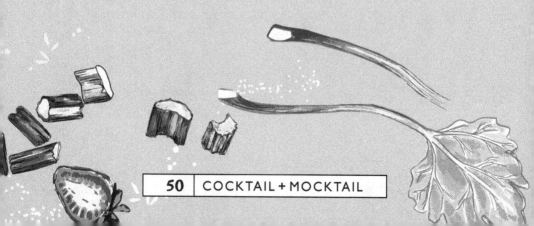

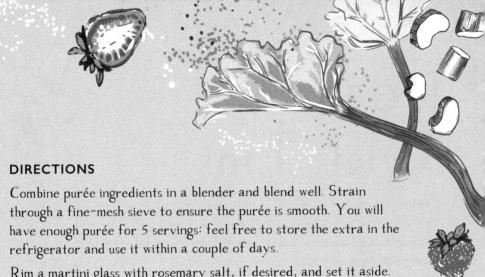

DIRECTIONS

Combine purée ingredients in a blender and blend well. Strain through a fine-mesh sieve to ensure the purée is smooth. You will have enough purée for 5 servings; feel free to store the extra in the refrigerator and use it within a couple of days.

Rim a martini glass with rosemary salt, if desired, and set it aside.

To make a cocktail, combine the rosemary rum, rosemary syrup, purée, and lemon juice in a glass canning jar.

To make a mocktail, combine the rosemary tea, rosemary syrup, purée, and lemon juice in a glass canning jar.

Fill the jar ⅔ full of ice, cap, and shake hard for 20 seconds. Strain the liquid off the ice and pour it into the martini glass, being careful not to disturb the salt rim. Top with cayenne tincture (for a cocktail) or cayenne vinegar (for a mocktail), if desired.

Garnish with a sprig of fresh rosemary and a ribbon of rhubarb threaded onto a cocktail pick, if desired.

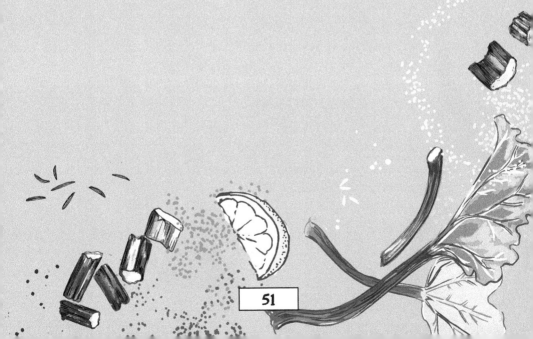

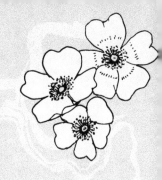

ROSY Tulsi-Tini

The perfect pre-dinner cocktail or mocktail with a calming adaptogen twist, this botanical martini is not only tasty but quite beautiful as well. Enjoy in a martini glass rimmed with rose petal sugar.

INGREDIENTS

2 fl oz (60 mL) tulsi vodka
(or cooled tulsi tea)

½ fl oz (15 mL) rose petal syrup

½ fl oz (15 mL) dry wild vermouth
(omit for a mocktail and increase tulsi tea by ½ fl oz)

2 tsp (10 mL) freshly squeezed lemon juice

10 drops rose petal syrup (optional)

Rose petal sugar for rimming (optional)

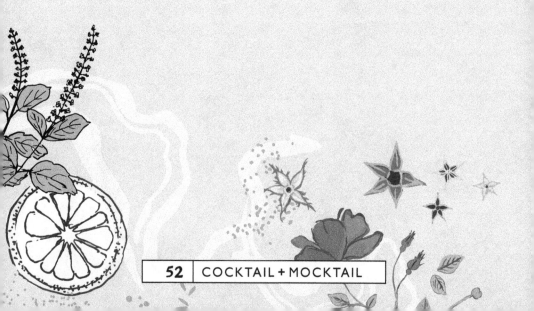

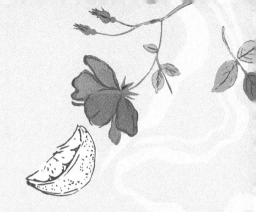

DIRECTIONS

Rim a martini glass with rose petal sugar, if desired, and set it aside.

To make a cocktail, combine the tulsi vodka, rose petal syrup, vermouth, and lemon juice in a glass canning jar.

To make a mocktail, combine the tulsi tea, rose petal syrup, and lemon juice (omitting the vermouth) in a glass canning jar.

Fill the jar ⅔ full of ice, cap, and shake hard for 20 seconds. Strain the liquid off the ice and pour it into the martini glass, being careful not to disturb the sugar rim.

Using a pipette, place a small amount of rose petal syrup in the bottom of the glass to give it a lovely pink coloring at the bottom, if desired.

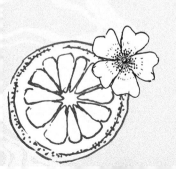

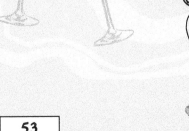

SPRING CLEAN
CHAI

Not quite ready to give winter chai up? Thankfully you don't have to! Filled with liver-supportive alterative herbs and tasty spices, this spring coffee alternative is a lovely mocktail for your morning, afternoon, or evening. Enjoy in a mug with a sprinkle of cinnamon and nutmeg as garnish.

INGREDIENTS

8 fl oz (240 mL) milk (dairy or non-dairy)

1 tbsp (15 mL) Liver Lover Syrup (ingredients below)

1-2 tbsp (15-30 mL) Chai Spice Syrup (ingredients below)

½ tsp (2.5 mL) vanilla extract

Sprinkle of cinnamon and nutmeg for garnish (optional)

LIVER LOVER SYRUP:

½ tbsp dandelion root

½ tbsp burdock root

½ tbsp rosehip

8 fl oz (240 mL) water

4 fl oz (120 mL) honey (or other sweetener)

CHAI SPICE SYRUP:

1½ cinnamon sticks

10 whole cloves

2 inches fresh ginger, minced

2 cardamom pods, crushed

8 fl oz (240 mL) water

4 fl oz (120 mL) honey (or other sweetener)

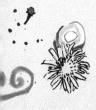

DIRECTIONS

To make each syrup, combine herbs and water in two separate small saucepans. Bring the mixture in each saucepan to a boil and then immediately lower the heat to a simmer. Simmer the mixture in each saucepan until the water level has reduced by half (approximately 4 fl oz (120 mL)). Remove each saucepan from the heat and allow the mixtures to cool. Strain each mixture through a fine-mesh sieve and compost herbs, reserving each finished liquid in separate clean bowls. Add honey (or other sweetener) to each bowl, and stir to thoroughly combine. Transfer the finished syrups to labeled glass bottles, and store in the refrigerator for up to 2 weeks.

To make the chai, add the milk to a small saucepan and heat over medium heat until the mixture begins to steam.

Immediately remove from heat and stir in syrups and vanilla before transferring to a heatproof mug.

Garnish with a sprinkle of cinnamon and nutmeg, if desired.

Spring Dandy
WHISKEY SOUR

Enjoy this classic whiskey sour with a springtime botanical twist. Strawberry, dandelion, and rhubarb—three spring plants that grow in abundance during this season—meet up for this sweet, yet sour cocktail that will give your body the jump-start it needs after winter. Enjoy in a rocks glass garnished with a fresh strawberry.

INGREDIENTS

2 fl oz (60 mL) strawberry bourbon

1 fl oz (30 mL) dandelion flower syrup

½ fl oz (15 mL) rhubarb vinegar

Fresh strawberry for garnish (optional)

DIRECTIONS

Combine all ingredients, except garnish, in a glass canning jar.

Fill the jar ⅔ full of ice, cap, and shake hard for 20 seconds. Strain the liquid off the ice and pour it into a rocks glass.

Garnish with a fresh strawberry, sliced halfway up the center and attached to the edge of the glass, if desired.

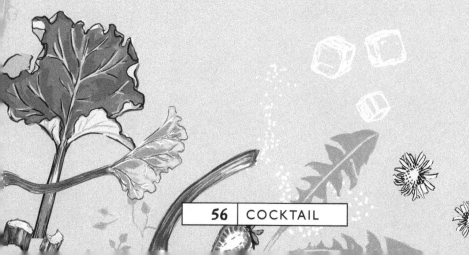

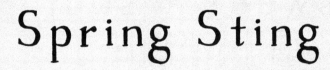

Spring Sting

Nettle is an early spring plant that is packed full of vitamins and minerals, and while we highly recommend enjoying it throughout the day as an herbal tea, feel free to reserve a bit for a refreshing afternoon delight. Enjoy this cocktail or mocktail over ice in a collins glass.

INGREDIENTS

2 fl oz (60 mL) cooled nettle tea

2 fl oz (60 mL) vodka (omit for a mocktail and add an extra 4 fl oz (120 mL) of carbonated water)

1 fl oz (30 mL) ginger syrup

½ fl oz (15 mL) freshly squeezed lemon juice

2 fl oz (60 mL) carbonated water, chilled

DIRECTIONS

Fill a collins glass half full with ice and set it aside.

To make a cocktail, combine the nettle tea, vodka, ginger syrup, and lemon juice in a glass canning jar.

To make a mocktail, combine the nettle tea, ginger syrup, and lemon juice in a glass canning jar.

Fill the jar ⅔ full of ice, cap, and shake hard for 20 seconds. Strain the liquid off the ice and into the collins glass.

Top with chilled carbonated water and gently stir to combine.

sweet + sour
GIMLET

The sour flavor helps to stimulate digestion and the cleansing processes in the body. Thankfully, it's easy to incorporate the sour flavor into your spring drinks along with a hint of sweetness to create a well-rounded, enjoyable drink. Enjoy this cocktail in a coupe glass and garnish with a fresh lilac or elderflower sprig.

INGREDIENTS

2 fl oz (60 mL) elderflower gin

2 fl oz (60 mL) grapefruit juice

½ fl oz (15 mL) lilac syrup

½ fl oz (15 mL) freshly squeezed lime juice

Fresh lilac or elderflower sprig for garnish (optional)

DIRECTIONS

Combine all ingredients, except garnish, in a glass canning jar.

Fill the jar ⅔ full of ice, cap, and shake hard for 20 seconds. Strain the liquid off the ice and pour it into a coupe glass.

Garnish with a fresh lilac or elderflower sprig, if desired.

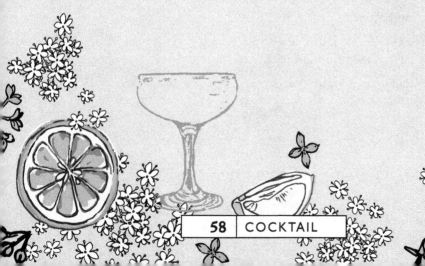

violet fizz

Simple, subtle, and tasty. That is the beauty of some mixed drink recipes, and this violet fizz is no exception. Enjoy as a cocktail or a mocktail in a rocks glass over ice with a garnish of fresh violet flowers. And to make this drink even more fancy, here's an additional garnish idea: use ice cubes with fresh violet flowers frozen inside for serving.

INGREDIENTS

2 fl oz (60 mL) violet vodka (or cooled violet tea)

¾ fl oz (20 mL) simple syrup

¾ fl oz (20 mL) freshly squeezed lemon juice

10 drops orange bitters (or orange vinegar)

Carbonated water to taste

10 drops violet syrup (optional)

Fresh violet flowers for garnish (optional)

DIRECTIONS

To make violet ice cubes for garnish, place a fresh violet flower in each cavity of an ice cube tray. Next, carefully fill each cavity of the tray with water. Don't worry about the violet floating to the top as this is expected. Place the ice cube tray in the freezer until fully frozen.

Fill a rocks glass with ice (or violet flower ice cubes) and set it aside.

To make a cocktail, combine the violet vodka, simple syrup, lemon juice, and orange bitters in a glass canning jar.

To make a mocktail, combine the violet tea, simple syrup, lemon juice, and orange vinegar in a glass canning jar.

Fill the jar ⅔ full of ice, cap, and shake hard for 20 seconds. Strain the liquid off the ice and pour over the ice in the rocks glass.

Slowly pour carbonated water over the ice.

Using a pipette, place a small amount of violet syrup in the bottom of the glass to give it a lovely purple coloring at the bottom, if desired.

Garnish the top with fresh violet flowers, if desired, add a straw for sipping, and serve.

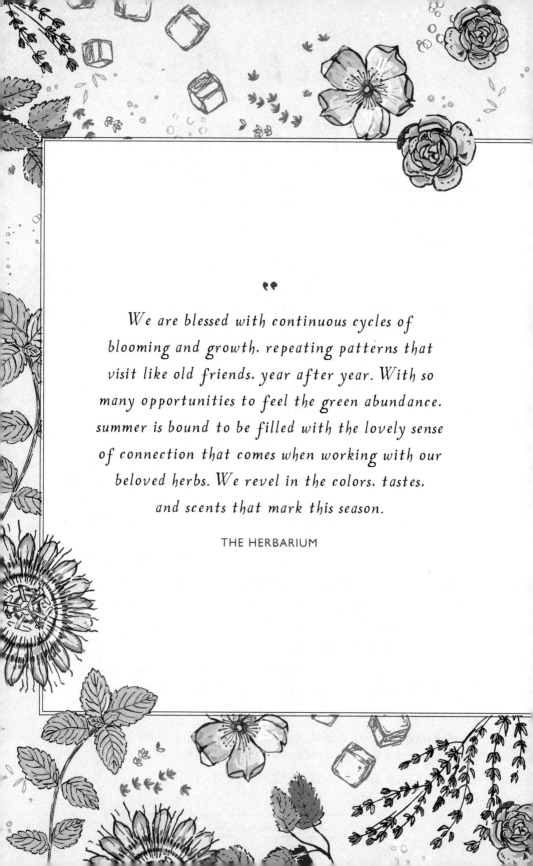

> *We are blessed with continuous cycles of blooming and growth, repeating patterns that visit like old friends, year after year. With so many opportunities to feel the green abundance, summer is bound to be filled with the lovely sense of connection that comes when working with our beloved herbs. We revel in the colors, tastes, and scents that mark this season.*

THE HERBARIUM

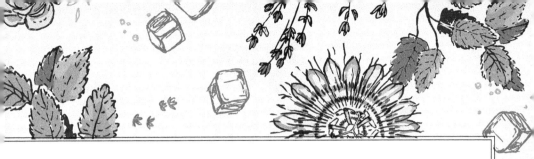

CHAPTER FOUR

SUMMER BOTANICAL MIXED DRINKS

As the summer sun beats down, we find ourselves craving cooling, refreshing drinks to provide a thirst-quenching respite. Shaken or stirred, these mixed drink recipes shine for nearly any occasion—whether you're attending a festive pool party or listening to the sound of cicadas from your porch swing.

When sourcing these ingredients, consider visiting your farmers market (or garden!) for the freshest seasonal herbs and fruits, including raspberries, watermelon, lemon balm, and thyme. Take a country drive with the windows down to sniff out some wild peppermint, or grab your foraging basket to pick juicy blueberries. Sip on summer as you count butterflies and ponder the magic of lightning bugs.

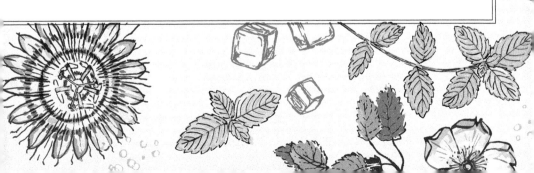

BERRY HERBY
— *B E L L I N I* —

There's something so perfect about the combination of strawberry and thyme. The flavor calls to mind a summer afternoon in the South. Combine this with some refreshing bubbly in a champagne flute, martini glass, coupe glass, or glass jar, and you've got yourself a tasty little pick-me-up cocktail or mocktail perfect for brunch, lunch, or an after-dinner treat. Enjoy along with fresh strawberries and fresh thyme sprigs as garnish.

INGREDIENTS

3 tbsp (45 mL) Strawberry Thyme Purée (ingredients below)

4 fl oz (120 mL) dry sparkling white wine, chilled (or carbonated water, chilled)

Fresh strawberries and fresh thyme sprig for garnish (optional)

STRAWBERRY THYME PURÉE:

2 cups ripe strawberries

3 tbsp fresh thyme

1 fl oz (30 mL) freshly squeezed lemon juice

2 fl oz (60 mL) simple syrup

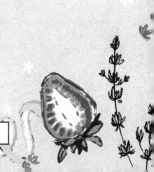

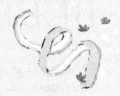

DIRECTIONS

Combine purée ingredients in a blender and blend well. Strain through a fine-mesh sieve to ensure the purée is smooth. You will have enough purée for 5 servings; feel free to store the extra in the refrigerator and use it within a couple of days.

Carefully add the purée to a small glass. Champagne flutes, martini and coupe glasses, and even jelly canning jars work well.

To make a cocktail, pour chilled sparkling wine over the purée. Stir gently to combine.

To make a mocktail, pour chilled carbonated water over the purée. Stir gently to combine.

Garnish with a cocktail pick or skewer layered with fresh strawberries and fresh sprigs of thyme placed between the berries and woven around the skewer, if desired.

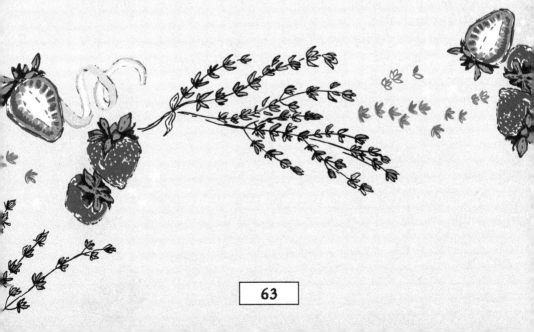

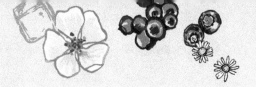

BLUE *Althaea* DELIGHT

This cooling, moistening botanical drink has a subtly sweet yet
tart flavor that is perfect for warm days of the year. Packed with
antioxidant goodness, you'll be reaching for this delicious mocktail
again and again. Enjoy in a collins glass over ice.

INGREDIENTS

1 handful fresh blueberries

6 fl oz (180 mL) cooled marshmallow root or flower tea

1½ fl oz (45 mL) anise hyssop syrup (or anise seed or licorice root
syrup)

½ fl oz (15 mL) freshly squeezed lime juice

2 dashes (20 drops) chamomile bitters (or chamomile glycerite)

DIRECTIONS

Fill a collins glass with ice and set it aside.

Muddle a handful of blueberries in a glass canning jar by pressing them
against the side of the jar with the back of a spoon to release their
juices before adding marshmallow tea and anise hyssop syrup to the
fruit. Stir to combine.

Pour over the ice in the collins glass, and top with chamomile bitters
(or chamomile glycerite for a totally alcohol-free option) before
stirring gently to combine.

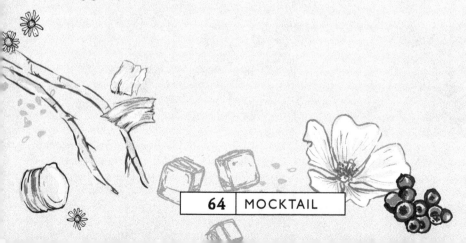

Calming Watermelon Spritzer

Lemon balm leaf, with its lemony flavor, and tulsi, with its hint of mint, are a lovely match for the sweet taste and vibrant color of watermelon in this hydrating, calming mocktail, making it a perfectly guiltless and refreshing drink. Enjoy in a collins glass over chilled watermelon cubes with a garnish of fresh lemon balm or tulsi leaves.

INGREDIENTS

6 fresh tulsi leaves

6 tbsp watermelon

½ fl oz (15 mL) lemon balm syrup

½ fl oz (15 mL) freshly squeezed lemon juice

8 fl oz (240 mL) carbonated water

Fresh watermelon cubes and fresh lemon balm or tulsi leaves for garnish (optional)

DIRECTIONS

Combine fresh tulsi leaves and watermelon together in a blender and blend until a purée forms. If you prefer, you can strain the purée through a fine-mesh sieve to separate the juice from the pulp.

Add a few small chilled watermelon cubes to a collins glass, if desired, and set it aside.

Combine the purée (or the juice) along with the lemon balm syrup and lemon juice into a glass canning jar.

Fill the jar ⅔ full of ice, cap, and shake hard for 20 seconds. Strain the liquid off the ice and pour it into the collins glass. Top with carbonated water, and stir gently to combine.

Garnish with a few fresh lemon balm or tulsi leaves, if desired.

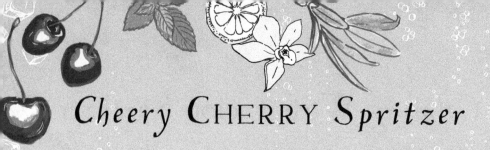

Cheery CHERRY Spritzer

This sparkling cheery cherry mocktail has a beautiful red color and a splash of uplifting nervines. Enjoy in a collins glass along with a lemon wheel and fresh sage or mint as garnish.

INGREDIENTS

8 fl oz (240 mL) carbonated water

2 fl oz (60 mL) cherry shrub

½ fl oz (15 mL) vanilla syrup

½ fl oz (15 mL) freshly squeezed lemon juice

10 drops lemon balm glycerite (or lemon balm vinegar)

10 drops milky oat glycerite (or milky oat vinegar)

Fresh sliced lemon wheel and fresh sage or mint leaves for garnish (optional)

DIRECTIONS

Fill a collins glass ⅓ full with crushed ice.

Combine all ingredients, except garnish, in the glass. Stir gently to combine.

Garnish with a fresh lemon slice and fresh sage or mint leaves, if desired.

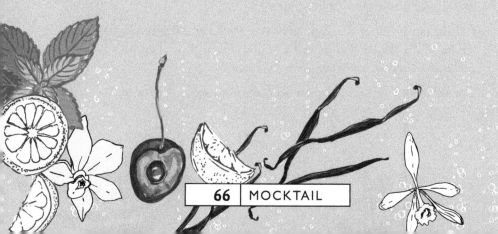

FRUITY FIZZ

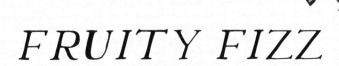

With its relaxing nervine and bitter digestive support, you'll feel good while sipping this summer mocktail to calm the mind and warm the digestive system. Enjoy in a collins glass with a garnish of fresh sliced peach and/or plum.

INGREDIENTS

6 fl oz (180 mL) fruit-flavored kombucha or water kefir (or carbonated water)

½–1 fl oz (15–30 mL) ginger syrup (plus more for pipetting, if desired)

60 drops nervine tincture (or nervine glycerite) of choice: skullcap, lemon balm, catnip, passionflower, linden, California poppy, etc.

Fresh sliced peaches and/or plums for garnish (optional)

DIRECTIONS

Fill a collins glass with a few ice cubes. Slice a fresh peach and/or plum thinly and wedge a few slices between the ice and the side of the glass, if desired.

Top the ice cubes with kombucha or water kefir (or carbonated water for a totally alcohol-free option), ginger syrup, and nervine tincture (or nervine glycerite for a totally alcohol-free option). Gently stir to combine.

Using a pipette, feel free to place extra ginger syrup in the bottom of the glass to give it a lovely yellow color and an extra hit of spicy sweetness.

Garnish with remaining fruit slices, if desired.

GARDEN MINT
—Old Fashioned—

This summery old fashioned highlights several cooling mint-family garden friends for a flavorful and stiff cocktail. Enjoy in a rocks glass over ice and garnish with a fresh mint sprig or two!

INGREDIENTS

2 fl oz (60 mL) mint bourbon

½ fl oz (15 mL) lemon balm syrup

½ tsp (2.5 mL) skullcap or wood betony tincture

Fresh mint sprig for garnish (optional)

DIRECTIONS

Fill a rocks glass with ice.

Add bourbon, syrup, and tincture to the glass, and stir to combine.

Garnish with a fresh mint sprig, if desired.

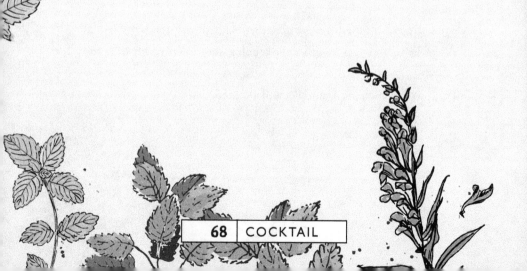

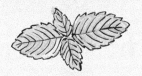

Kentucky Mint
REFRESHER

A classic summer mixed drink recipe with an extra pop of minty goodness to make it all the more refreshing. Not only that, but mint (both peppermint and spearmint) is a great way to soothe digestion, cool the body, and calm inflammation. Choose one mint or use them both to make this popular cocktail even more botanically complex! Enjoy in a classic julep cup or a collins glass over crushed ice with a fresh mint sprig for garnish.

INGREDIENTS

5 fresh mint leaves

2 fl oz (60 mL) mint bourbon

1 fl oz (30 mL) mint syrup

1 fl oz (30 mL) water or carbonated water

Fresh mint sprig for garnish (optional)

DIRECTIONS

Begin by muddling five fresh mint leaves in the bottom of a mint julep cup or collins glass by pressing them against the sides of the glass with the back of a spoon. Fill the glass ½ full of crushed ice.

Add the remainder of the ingredients, except garnish, to the glass and gently stir, carefully avoiding mixing the muddled mint leaves into the ice. You want them to remain toward the bottom of the glass for color.

Fill the glass with additional crushed ice, and carefully stir once more.

Garnish with a sprig of fresh mint, if desired.

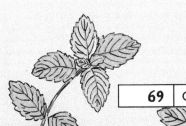

Late Summer
WELLNESS CORDIAL

This late summer cordial recipe is packed with tonic, lymphatic, and immune-supportive herbs that will help to bolster the immune system and encourage wellness as summer transitions to back-to-school season and the forthcoming cold and flu season. Note: this recipe takes 4-6 weeks to prepare.

Yield: 20 fl oz, or 10 servings (2 fl oz each)

INGREDIENTS

½ cup tulsi

¼ cup milky oat

¼ cup burdock root

⅛ cup calendula

⅛ cup astragalus root

1-inch piece fresh ginger, minced

16 fl oz (480 mL) whiskey (or enough to fill jar)

8 fl oz (240 mL) honey (or other sweetener)

DIRECTIONS

Combine all ingredients, except honey, in a quart-sized glass jar. Place a piece of natural waxed paper between the jar and lid, cap, and label the jar. Place the jar in a warm, dark location for 4-6 weeks. Invert or roll jar in hands a few times every 1-2 days to mix. Mixture may look foamy after mixing.

When time is up, strain the mixture through a fine-mesh sieve. Compost the herbs and transfer the liquid to a clean glass jar. Add honey. Cap and label the jar, and give it a good shake to mix the honey into the liquid. Store the cordial in a cool, dark location for 1-2 years.

To serve, pour 2 fl oz (60 mL) in a cordial glass and sip on its own, add to a heatproof mug of just-boiled water for a quick and easy hot toddy, or add to a collins glass and top with carbonated water, kombucha, or water kefir for a cool, fizzy pick-me-up.

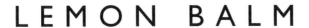

LEMON BALM
— *MARTINI* —

What to do with all that extra lemon balm during the summer? Make martinis, that's what! This dry martini packs a flavorful punch and will cheer your taste buds and emotions all at the same time. Enjoy this cocktail in a martini glass with a sprig of fresh lemon balm as garnish.

INGREDIENTS

5 fresh lemon balm leaves

2 fl oz (60 mL) gin

½ fl oz (15 mL) simple syrup

½ fl oz (15 mL) freshly squeezed lemon juice

Fresh sprig of lemon balm for garnish (optional)

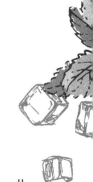

DIRECTIONS

Combine gin, simple syrup, lemon juice, and fresh lemon balm in a small blender and pulse until the leaves are roughly chopped.

Strain through a fine-mesh sieve. Compost herbs and pour liquid into a glass canning jar.

Fill the jar ⅔ full of ice, cap, and shake hard for 20 seconds. Strain the liquid off the ice and pour it into a martini glass.

Garnish with a sprig of fresh lemon balm, if desired.

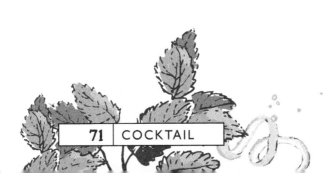

Minty *Rose* Mojito

Fresh peppermint is synonymous with mojitos. Add in some subtly sweet rose petal to the mix and you have yourself a perfect botanical combination that is cooling and soothing during the hot months of summer! Enjoy this cocktail in a rocks glass over ice with fresh mint leaves for garnish.

INGREDIENTS

1 fresh mint sprig (plus extra leaves for garnish)

2 fl oz (60 mL) peppermint rum

2 fl oz (60 mL) rose petal syrup

1 fl oz (30 mL) freshly squeezed lime juice

2 dashes (20 drops) motherwort bitters (or mugwort scotch)

Carbonated water (optional)

DIRECTIONS

Muddle the fresh mint sprig in the bottom of a rocks glass by pressing it against the glass with the back of a spoon to release its aromatics.

Add in the mint rum, rose petal syrup, and lime juice, and stir well.

Fill the glass with crushed ice and top with carbonated water, if desired. Top with 2 dashes of bitters.

Garnish with additional fresh mint leaves, if desired.

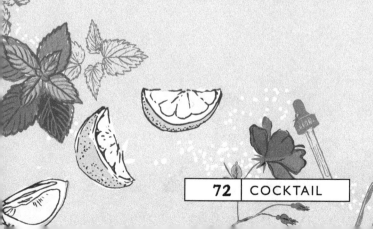

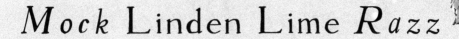

Mock Linden Lime *Razz*

This mocktail with a classic flavor combination has a botanical twist and is a lovely way to wind down after a long, stimulating day of fun in the sun! Linden lends its slightly sweet, moistening, heart-relaxing properties while raspberry offers some sweet antioxidants of its own. Followed up by the savory aroma of basil, this visually beautiful drink is a summer must-have. Enjoy in a rocks glass with a basil salt rim and fresh basil sprig as garnish.

INGREDIENTS

4 fresh raspberries

2 fl oz (60 mL) cooled linden flower tea

½ fl oz (15 mL) simple syrup

½ fl oz (15 mL) freshly squeezed lime juice

Basil salt for rimming (optional)

Fresh sprig of basil for garnish (optional)

DIRECTIONS

Rim a rocks glass with basil salt, if desired. Fill the glass with ice, being careful not to disturb the salt rim, and set it aside.

Muddle the raspberries in a glass canning jar by pressing them against the side of the jar with the back of a spoon to release their juices before adding cooled linden tea, simple syrup, and lime juice to the jar.

Fill the jar ⅔ full of ice, cap, and shake hard for 20 seconds. Strain the liquid off the ice and carefully pour it into the rocks glass, again being careful not to disturb the salt rim.

Garnish with a sprig of fresh basil, if desired.

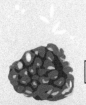
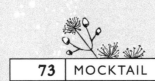
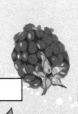
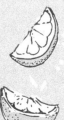

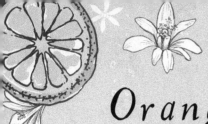
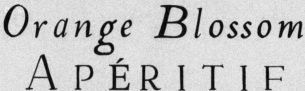

Orange Blossom
APÉRITIF

Apéritifs are traditionally served before meals to help stimulate the appetite and prepare the digestive system for the upcoming meal. This orange blossom apéritif recipe is a super simple, effervescent way to consume bitters, and it's inspired by the classic Italian aperol spritz. Enjoy this cocktail in a wine glass and garnish with an orange wheel.

INGREDIENTS

3 fl oz (90 mL) prosecco, chilled

1 fl oz (30 mL) carbonated water

1 tsp (5 mL) orange blossom water (store-bought)

2 dashes (20 drops) orange bitters

Fresh orange wheel for garnish (optional)

DIRECTIONS

Fill a wine glass with ice.

Combine all ingredients, except garnish, in the glass, and stir until well combined.

Garnish with a fresh orange wheel, if desired.

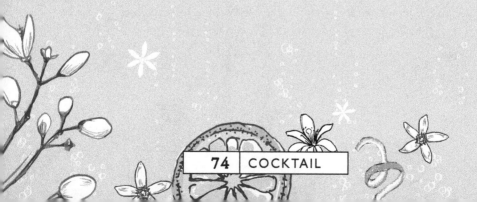

Pineapple Ginger
FROZEN DAIQUIRI

This tropical frozen daiquiri is the perfect poolside beverage to keep you cool on hot summer days. If you're not a fan of frozen drinks, feel free to skip the ice and top this mix with carbonated water after blending. Enjoy as a cocktail or mocktail in a martini glass rimmed with rose petal sugar and a pineapple wedge and mint leaves for garnish.

INGREDIENTS

2 fl oz (60 mL) pineapple juice

1 fl oz (30 mL) light rum (or cooled white tea)

1 fl oz (30 mL) ginger syrup

1 tsp (5 mL) freshly squeezed lemon juice

⅔ cup crushed ice

Rose petal sugar for rimming (optional)

Fresh peppermint leaves and a pineapple wedge for garnish (optional)

DIRECTIONS

Rim a martini glass with rose petal sugar, if desired, and set it aside.

To make a cocktail, add pineapple juice, rum, ginger syrup, lemon juice, and crushed ice to a blender.

To make a mocktail, add pineapple juice, white tea, ginger syrup, lemon juice, and crushed ice to a blender.

Pulse/blend the mixture on high for 30 seconds until smooth. Carefully pour into a martini glass, being careful not to disturb the sugar rim.

Garnish with fresh peppermint leaves and a pineapple wedge, if desired.

Pirate Paloma

You and your shipmates will love this spicy mixed drink that will transport you to a warm beach on a remote Caribbean island. This cocktail or mocktail can be enjoyed any time of the year but is especially lovely when you're missing the sun. Enjoy in a collins glass over ice and garnish with fresh grapefruit. Note that the spiced rum needs to be prepared 2 weeks ahead of time.

INGREDIENTS

2 fl oz (60 mL) Spiced Rum (or Herbal Chai) (ingredients below)

½ fl oz (15 mL) simple syrup

1 fl oz (30 mL) freshly squeezed grapefruit juice

½ fl oz (15 mL) freshly squeezed lime juice

Carbonated water

Fresh grapefruit peel for garnish (optional)

SPICED RUM OR HERBAL CHAI:

3 cinnamon sticks, crushed

1 star anise pod

20 whole cloves

4 inches fresh ginger, minced

3 cardamom pods, crushed

¼ tsp nutmeg powder

8 fl oz (240 mL) rum or boiled water

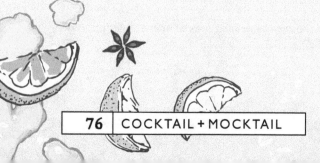

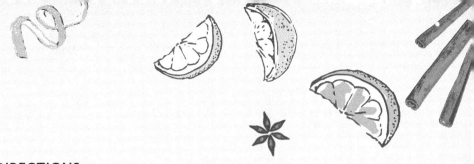

DIRECTIONS

To make spiced rum, combine all spiced rum ingredients in a glass canning jar. Place a piece of natural waxed paper between the jar and the lid and seal. Label the jar, shake, and place in a dark location for 2 weeks before straining through a fine-mesh sieve, composting herbs, and reserving spiced rum in a clean, labeled glass jar or bottle to be used within 1-2 years.

To make herbal chai, combine all ingredients in a glass canning jar and carefully add boiled water. Cap with a small plate or a lid to trap the steam and volatile oils inside the jar. Steep for 30-60 minutes before straining through a fine-mesh sieve, composting herbs, and reserving the herbal chai in a clean, labeled glass jar in the refrigerator to use within 24 hours. Extra chai may be used in a baking recipe or to sweeten and drink as is.

Fill a collins glass with ice. Wedge a strip of grapefruit peel between the ice and the glass, if desired, and set it aside.

To make a cocktail, combine the spiced rum, grapefruit and lime juices, and simple syrup in a glass canning jar.

To make a mocktail, combine the spiced chai, grapefruit and lime juices, and simple syrup in a glass canning jar.

Fill the jar ⅔ full of ice, cap, and shake hard for 20 seconds. Strain the liquid off the ice and pour over the ice in the collins glass. Top by slowly pouring carbonated water over the ice.

Garnish with another fresh grapefruit peel, if desired.

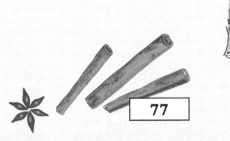

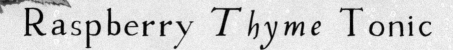

Raspberry *Thyme* Tonic

This light sweet and sour cocktail is refreshing and rejuvenating on a hot summer's day. Sip slowly as you perform a monotonous task or while relaxing on the front porch. Enjoy in a glass canning jar with a sprig of fresh thyme for garnish.

INGREDIENTS

¼ cup frozen raspberries

½ fl oz (15 mL) thyme vinegar

2 tsp (8g) cane sugar (or sugar alternative)

4 fl oz (120 mL) boiled water

1 fl oz (30 mL) vodka

4 fl oz (120 mL) carbonated water

Fresh sprig of thyme for garnish (optional)

DIRECTIONS

Place raspberries, vinegar, and sugar in a heatproof glass jar. Add boiled water and stir for a minute or so before setting the mixture aside to cool.

Once mixture is cool, fill a glass canning jar half full with ice, and set it aside.

Add the vodka to the glass canning jar with the raspberry mixture.

Fill the jar ⅔ full of ice, cap, and shake hard for 20 seconds. Strain the liquid off the ice and pour it into the glass canning jar with ice. Top with carbonated water.

Garnish with a sprig of thyme, if desired.

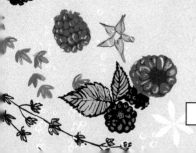

Really Rosy Faux Rosé

Fill your heart (and glass) with beauty and joy with this faux rosé mocktail, perfect for a festive celebration with friends or as a gentle pick-me-up when your emotions are feeling a little raw. Enjoy in a champagne glass with a rose petal sugar rim and fresh (or dried) rose petals for garnish.

INGREDIENTS

2 fl oz (60 mL) strong, cooled rose petal tea

½ fl oz (15 mL) rose petal syrup

2 fl oz (60 mL) carbonated water, chilled

Rose petal sugar for rimming (optional)

Fresh or dried rose petals for garnish (optional)

DIRECTIONS

Rim a champagne glass with rose petal syrup and rose petal sugar, if desired, and set it aside.

Combine chilled rose petal tea and rose petal syrup together and mix to combine. Carefully pour the mixture into the champagne glass without disturbing the rose petal sugar rim. Top with chilled carbonated water and gently stir to combine.

Garnish with a skewer of fresh rose petals or a dusting of dried crushed rose petals over the top of the drink, if desired.

RUM *to* BED

Savor the toasted sweet flavor of rum and the island notes of coconut while lavender and hops gently lull you to sleep. Enjoy this cocktail in a coupe glass and garnish with a sprinkling of powdered nutmeg.

INGREDIENTS

2 fl oz (60 mL) aged rum

4 fl oz (120 mL) Lavender-Infused Coconut Milk (ingredients below)

½ fl oz (15 mL) blackberry or elderberry syrup

2 tsp (10 mL) black currant liqueur (store-bought)

10 drops hops tincture

Powdered nutmeg for garnish (optional)

LAVENDER-INFUSED COCONUT MILK:

4 fl oz (120 mL) coconut milk

½ tsp lavender

DIRECTIONS

To make lavender-infused coconut milk, combine coconut milk and lavender flower bud in a small saucepan over low heat. As soon as the milk begins to steam, remove from heat and cover with a lid to steep for 10 minutes. Strain milk through a fine-mesh sieve. Compost the lavender and let the lavender-infused coconut milk cool.

Combine all ingredients, except nutmeg, in a glass canning jar.

Fill the jar ⅔ full of ice, cap, and shake hard for 20 seconds. Strain the liquid off the ice and pour it into a coupe glass.

Garnish with powdered nutmeg, if desired.

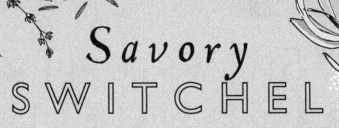

Savory SWITCHEL

This savory switchel has an herbaceous flavor that is suitable for any time of the year. You can use the Basic Botanical Vinegar recipe on page 22 and experiment with your favorite savory herbs, such as thyme, sage, nettle, and rosemary. While switchels are usually made as a healthy, hydrating nonalcoholic beverage, we've included a cocktail option for this one. Enjoy in a rocks glass over ice and garnish with a fresh sage leaf.

INGREDIENTS

1 fl oz (30 mL) thyme vodka (or cooled thyme tea)

1 fl oz (30 mL) simple syrup

1 fl oz (30 mL) botanical vinegar

2 fl oz (60 mL) carbonated water

Fresh sage leaf for garnish (optional)

DIRECTIONS

Fill a rocks glass with ice.

To make a cocktail, combine the thyme vodka, botanical vinegar, syrup, and carbonated water in the rocks glass, and stir to combine.

To make a mocktail, combine the thyme tea, botanical vinegar, syrup, and carbonated water in the rocks glass, and stir to combine.

Garnish with a fresh sage leaf, if desired.

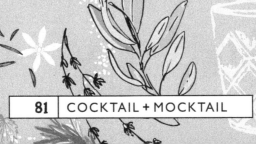

SHOWSTOPPER LIMONCELLO

This fun limoncello recipe is great to serve in front of an audience because it "magically" changes color from a purple-blue to a vibrant pink with the addition of lemon juice! Enjoy as a cocktail or mocktail over ice in a collins glass with fresh strawberries, blueberries, or a lemon slice for garnish.

Yield: 38 fl oz, or 4 servings (9.5 fl oz each)

INGREDIENTS

12 fl oz (360 mL) cooled violet tea (use 16 fl oz (480 mL) for a mocktail)

16 fl oz (480 mL) cooled Red Cabbage Decoction (ingredients below)

4 fl oz (120 mL) lemon vodka (omit for mocktail)

6 fl oz (180 mL) freshly squeezed lemon juice

Fresh strawberries, blueberries, or lemon slice for garnish (optional)

RED CABBAGE DECOCTION:

1 cup red cabbage leaves

16 fl oz (480 mL) water

½ cup (100 g) cane sugar (or sugar alternative)

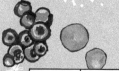

DIRECTIONS

Four hours before serving, prepare the cabbage decoction by boiling the cabbage leaves and water in a saucepan for 1 minute before removing the saucepan from heat, carefully straining the mixture through a fine-mesh sieve, and composting the plant material (or reserving it for later use). Transfer the reserved cabbage liquid into a clean saucepan. The liquid should be a purple-blue color. Add in ½ cup of sugar (or sugar alternative) and stir well to dissolve. Place this mixture in the refrigerator to cool completely.

Then, prepare the violet tea by adding 3 tbsp violet flower to a glass canning jar along with 12 fl oz boiling water. Cover and let infuse for 20 minutes, then cap and place in the refrigerator to chill.

When ready to serve, fill each collins glass ½ full of ice and set aside.

For cocktails, combine cabbage decoction, 12 fl oz (360 mL) violet tea, and lemon vodka in a large glass jar or pitcher and stir to combine.

For mocktails, combine cabbage decoction with 16 fl oz (480 mL) violet tea in a large glass jar or pitcher and stir to combine.

Pour cocktail or mocktail into individual collins glasses and garnish each with a strawberry, sliced halfway up the center and attached to the edge of the glasses, or toss a few fresh blueberries or a lemon slice into the glass, if desired.

When you're ready to impress your guests, give each of them a small bowl or cup filled with 3 tbsp (45 mL) lemon juice to pour into their glass. As soon as they pour it in and give it a gentle stir, it will shift from a purple-blue color to a vibrant red!

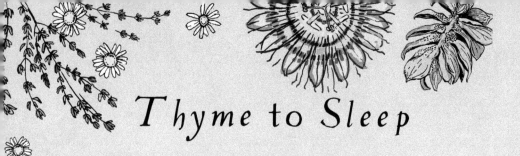

Thyme to Sleep

Hops and passionflower aren't the tastiest of sedative herbs—but paired with a thyme simple syrup you'll never know you've taken a helpful dose of these soporific sisters. Enjoy this cocktail in a rocks glass over ice with fresh lemon peel and a thyme sprig for garnish.

INGREDIENTS

1½ fl oz (45 mL) bourbon

¾ fl oz (20 mL) thyme syrup

3 dashes (30 drops) chamomile bitters

10 drops passionflower tincture

10 drops hops tincture

Fresh lemon peel and a sprig of thyme for garnish (optional)

DIRECTIONS

Add all ingredients, except garnish, to a rocks glass, fill with ice, and stir to combine.

Garnish with a fresh lemon peel and a sprig of fresh thyme, if desired.

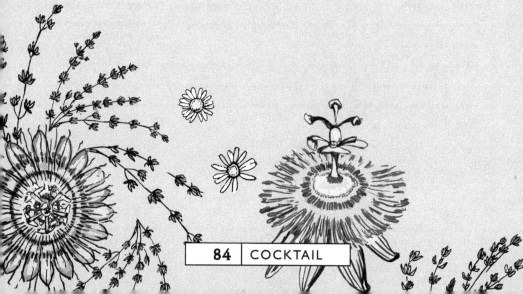

Tulsi Lime
MARGARITA

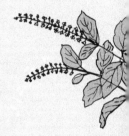

Lime juice and tulsi, also known as holy basil, are an incredibly refreshing combination for hot summer days. Because lime juice is a traditional ingredient in margaritas, this cocktail comes together beautifully with the addition of high-quality tequila. Enjoy in a rocks glass over ice with a salt rim and fresh lime wedge as garnish.

INGREDIENTS

2 sprigs fresh tulsi (optional but highly recommended!)

2 fl oz (60 mL) tequila

1 fl oz (30 mL) tulsi syrup

2 fl oz (60 mL) freshly squeezed lime juice

Salt for rimming (optional)

Fresh lime wedge for garnish (optional)

DIRECTIONS

Rim a rocks glass with lime juice and salt, if desired.

Muddle the fresh tulsi sprigs in the bottom of your salt-rimmed glass by pressing them against the glass with the back of a spoon to release their aromatics, being careful not to disturb the salt rim. (This step is optional and you can skip it if you don't have fresh tulsi. However, it really helps highlight the tulsi flavor.)

Fill the glass with ice and set it aside.

Combine the tequila, tulsi syrup, and lime juice in a glass canning jar.

Fill the jar ⅔ full of ice, cap, and shake hard for 20 seconds. Strain the liquid off the ice and pour it into the rocks glass, again being careful not to disturb the salt rim.

Garnish with a fresh lime wedge, if desired.

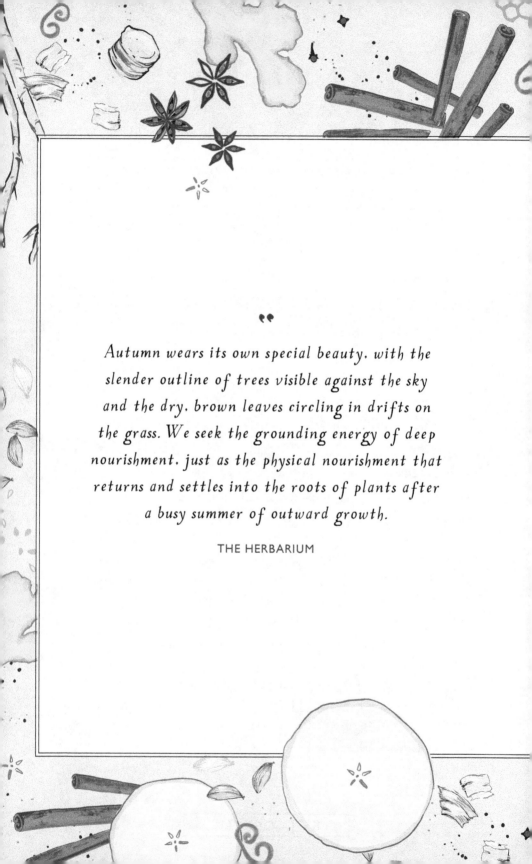

"

Autumn wears its own special beauty, with the slender outline of trees visible against the sky and the dry, brown leaves circling in drifts on the grass. We seek the grounding energy of deep nourishment, just as the physical nourishment that returns and settles into the roots of plants after a busy summer of outward growth.

THE HERBARIUM

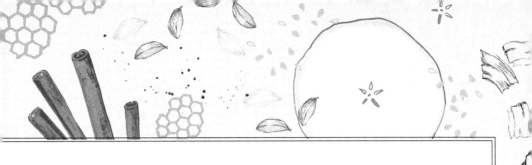

CHAPTER FIVE

AUTUMN BOTANICAL MIXED DRINKS

As the air gains a chilly edge and the leaves begin to fall, we feel the call to turn inward in preparation for colder days ahead. We fill our pantries with warming spices and nourishing roots, fruits, and late-season herbs from the fall harvest to support our families through winter. On afternoon walks we might gather brilliant red hawthorn and sumac berries, vitamin C-rich rose hips, maitake mushroom, dandelion root, and burdock root as we take in the fleeting beauty of this season.

Wrapped in cozy blankets, we find ourselves craving mulled cider, chai latte, and other autumnal favorites rich in the warming flavors of cinnamon, cardamom, and ginger. These botanical mixed drinks are perfect for nearly any crisp-weather outing. Feel the warmth move through your body as you traipse through the pumpkin patch or sip silently by the flickering fire.

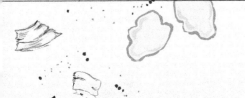
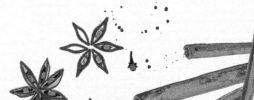

AFTER-DINNER
Hawthorn Elixir

This after-dinner elixir will not only help to encourage post-meal digestion, but it supports a happy, healthy heart as well. Infused with the flavors of the harvest season, this elixir will be your go-to autumn digestif for years to come! Enjoy this cocktail in a cordial glass by itself, in a heatproof mug with some hot water for a warm drink, or in a collins class with some carbonated water, kombucha, or water kefir for a cool drink. Note: this recipe takes 4-6 weeks to prepare.

Yield: 24 fl oz, or 12 servings (2 fl oz each)

INGREDIENTS

½ cup hawthorn berry

8 fl oz (240 mL) pear juice (or apple juice)

¼ cup chamomile

1 pear, chopped

2 tsp fresh ginger, minced

4 fl oz (120 mL) honey (or other sweetener)

16 fl oz (480 mL) brandy

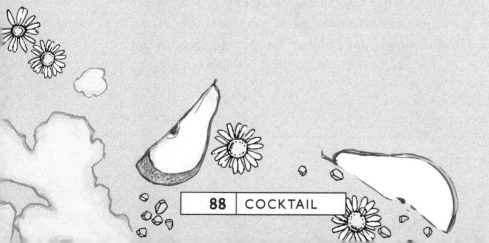

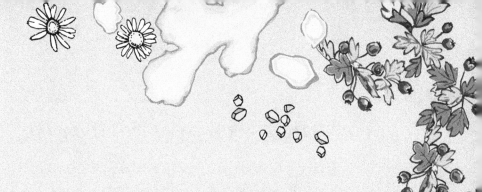

DIRECTIONS

Place hawthorn berry in a stainless steel saucepan and cover with pear or apple juice. Simmer over low heat for 15–20 minutes, and then transfer to a quart-sized glass canning jar and add the chamomile, pear, and ginger. Add honey and brandy and stir well to combine. Place a piece of natural waxed paper between the jar and lid, cover, and set aside in a warm, dark location for 4–6 weeks to infuse. Invert or roll jar in hands a few times every 1–2 days to mix.

When time is up, strain the contents of the jar through a fine-mesh sieve. Compost the herbs and reserve the liquid in a labeled glass jar. Store the elixir in a cool, dark location for up to 1 year.

To serve, pour 2 fl oz (60 mL) in a cordial glass and sip on its own, add to a heatproof mug of just-boiled water for a quick and easy hot toddy, or add to a collins glass and top with carbonated water, kombucha, or water kefir for a cool, fizzy pick-me-up.

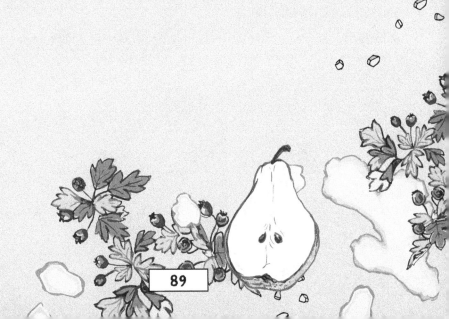

Autumn Apple Sangria

Sangrias are a great party drink any time of the year, tweaked to include seasonal spices and fruits. Apples are plentiful throughout autumn, so wow your guests with this delicious apple-spiced sangria that is sure to complement any fall gathering. Enjoy this cocktail in a wine glass.

Yield: 57 fl oz, or 9 servings (6 fl oz each)

INGREDIENTS

1 bottle (750 mL) Sweet Spiced Wine recipe (see recipe on p. 138, or use any fruity red wine)

8 fl oz (240 mL) apple juice

4 fl oz (120 mL) cinnamon liqueur

1 cup fresh red apple, sliced

1 cup fresh green apple, sliced

20 fl oz (600 mL) ginger beer (or carbonated water)

DIRECTIONS

Combine wine, apple juice, cinnamon liqueur, and fresh apples in a pitcher and stir well.

Refrigerate 2 hours or until ready to serve. Top with ginger beer (or carbonated water) before serving in wine glasses.

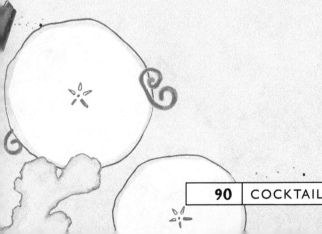

BITTER UNDERGROUND

Some of our favorite herbal roots make up this earthy, grounding cocktail for bitter lovers. It's perfect as an apéritif before meals. Enjoy in a martini glass.

INGREDIENTS

3 fl oz (90 mL) ginger tea

1½ tsp (7.5 mL) honey

1 fl oz (30 mL) vodka

1 fl oz (30 mL) brandy

1½ tsp (7.5 mL) burdock root tincture

½ tsp (2.5 mL) angelica root tincture

DIRECTIONS

Combine ginger tea and honey. Mix well and allow to completely cool.

Combine all ingredients in a quart-sized glass jar with ice.

Fill the jar ⅔ full of ice, cap, and shake hard for 20 seconds. Strain the liquid off the ice and pour it into a martini glass.

Bloody
ROSEMARY

Traditionally a morning drink, this botanical twist on a bloody mary can be enjoyed morning or evening. It's a smidge on the sweet side— herbal bitters are necessary to bring this colorful drink into the perfect balance. Note that orange liqueur or syrup can be substituted for the blood orange liqueur or syrup. Enjoy as a cocktail or mocktail in a rocks glass over ice with a fresh rosemary sprig for garnish.

INGREDIENTS

1 blood orange wheel, sliced ¼-inch thick from the midsection of the fruit

1 sprig fresh rosemary

1 fl oz (30 mL) gin (or cooled rosemary tea)

1 fl oz (30 mL) blood orange liqueur (or blood orange syrup)

2 tsp (10 mL) rosemary syrup

½ fl oz (15 mL) freshly squeezed lemon juice

½ fl oz (15 mL) freshly squeezed blood orange juice

3 dashes (30 drops) orange bitters (or orange vinegar)

Additional fresh rosemary sprig for garnish (optional)

DIRECTIONS

Fill a rocks glass with ice. Wedge a fresh blood orange slice between the ice and the side of the glass, and set the glass aside.

Muddle a rosemary sprig in a glass canning jar by pressing it against the glass with the back of a spoon to release its aromatics.

To make a cocktail, combine the gin, blood orange liqueur, rosemary syrup, lemon and blood orange juices, and orange bitters with the muddled rosemary in the glass canning jar.

To make a mocktail, combine the rosemary tea, blood orange syrup, rosemary syrup, lemon and blood orange juices, and orange vinegar with the muddled rosemary in the glass canning jar.

Fill the jar ⅔ full of ice, cap, and shake hard for 20 seconds. Strain the liquid off the ice and pour it into the rocks glass.

Garnish with an additional rosemary sprig nestled between the ice and the side of the glass, if desired.

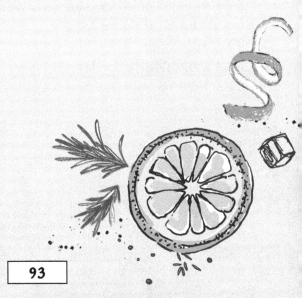

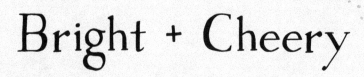

Bright + Cheery

This herb-infused cocktail is loosely based on the dark and stormy—a close cousin to the moscow mule. The addition of hawthorn and goldenrod bring a note of cheer and sunshine, and this cocktail will brighten up any dark or stormy day. Enjoy in a collins glass over ice with a fresh lime wedge for garnish.

INGREDIENTS

2 fl oz (60 mL) goldenrod rum

4 fl oz (120 mL) cooled ginger tea

1½ fl oz (45 mL) hawthorn berry syrup

½ fl oz (15 mL) freshly squeezed lime juice

Fresh lime wedge for garnish (optional)

DIRECTIONS

Fill a collins glass ⅔ full with crushed ice and set it aside.

Combine all ingredients, except garnish, in a glass canning jar.

Fill the jar ⅔ full of ice, cap, and shake hard for 20 seconds. Strain the liquid off the ice and pour it over the ice in the collins glass.

Garnish with a fresh lime wedge, if desired.

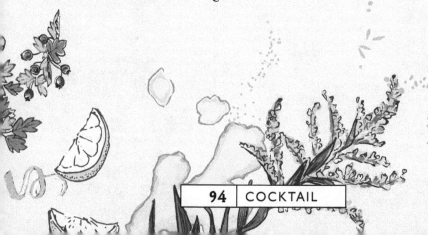

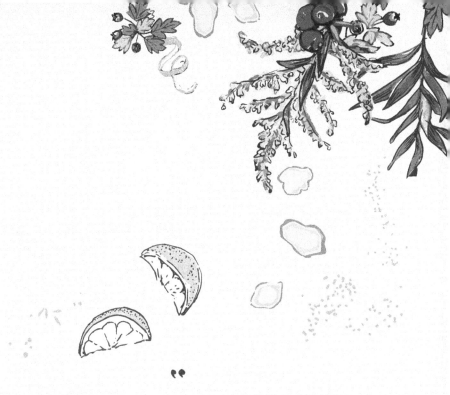

Goldenrod begins to grace fields and roadsides with its brilliant yellow flowers right at the peak of summer—as if each blossom is reflecting the warmth and joy of sunshiney days. Goldenrod carries that summer radiance all the way into fall, when most other flowers have said goodbye for the year. Bottling up that joy by making a goldenrod-infused spirit is such a nice way to brighten up the darker days of fall and winter.

LISA OLSON, RH(AHG) COURSE DEVELOPMENT DIRECTOR AT HERBAL ACADEMY

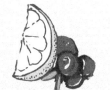

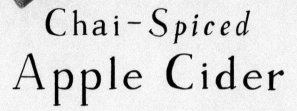

Chai-Spiced Apple Cider

Packed to the brim with warming herbs like cloves, cardamom, peppercorns, and cinnamon, this apple cider cocktail or mocktail is more herbal tonic than festive beverage, and we'll gladly enjoy the benefits of both with this recipe! Enjoy in a heatproof mug.

Yield: 32-38 fl oz, or 5-6 servings (6 fl oz each)

INGREDIENTS

16 fl oz (480 mL) Chai Concentrate (ingredients below)

16 fl oz (480 mL) apple cider

6 fl oz (180 mL) spiced rum (optional)

Star anise pods for garnish (optional)

CHAI CONCENTRATE:

6 cardamom pods, crushed (adjust to taste)

6 whole peppercorns

4 whole cloves

2 star anise pods

1-inch piece fresh ginger, minced

3 cinnamon sticks

20 fl oz (600 mL) water

2 black tea bags (or 2 tsp looseleaf black tea)

½ fl oz (15 mL) honey (or other sweetener)

2 tsp (10 mL) vanilla extract

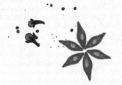

DIRECTIONS

Prepare chai concentrate by combining the cardamom, peppercorns, cloves, star anise, ginger, cinnamon, and water into a small saucepan and bring to a boil over high heat.

Once boiling, immediately reduce the heat to medium-low, cover, and simmer for 20 minutes.

Remove from heat, add the black tea and honey, cover, and allow to steep for 5 minutes. Any longer and the black tea may become bitter tasting.

Strain the mixture through a fine-mesh sieve and compost the herbs. Add the vanilla extract and stir to combine. Reserve the liquid and use right away or refrigerate for up to 24 hours before making the cocktail or mocktail.

For a cocktail, combine spiced rum, chai concentrate, and apple cider in a large crockpot set to warm.

For a mocktail, combine chai concentrate and apple cider in a large crockpot set to warm.

Serve in heatproof mugs once heated, garnishing with star anise pods, if desired.

Store leftover mixture in the refrigerator and use within 24 hours.

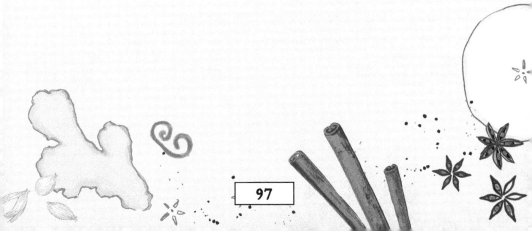

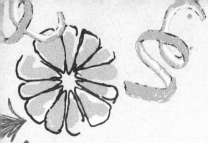
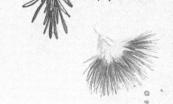

GIN WIZ

Rosemary can help boost focus and memory, and it contains carnosic acid, an antioxidant that can fight off damage from free radicals. Mimosa is one of our favorite relaxing nervines that helps to release tension. Finally, pink is thought to have a calming effect, and this pink cocktail is as good to look at as it is to drink! Enjoy in a collins glass over ice with a fresh rosemary or thyme sprig or rose petals for garnish.

INGREDIENTS

1 fl oz (30 mL) gin

2 fl oz (60 mL) rosemary syrup

6 fl oz (180 mL) pink grapefruit juice

½ fl oz (15 mL) freshly squeezed lime juice

10 drops mimosa tincture

Fresh rosemary or thyme sprig or rose petals for garnish (optional)

DIRECTIONS

Fill a collins glass ⅓ full of crushed ice and set it aside.

Combine gin, rosemary syrup, pink grapefruit juice, and lime juice in a glass canning jar.

Fill the jar ⅔ full of ice, cap, and shake hard for 20 seconds. Strain the liquid off the ice and pour it into the collins glass.

Add 10 drops of mimosa tincture and stir to combine.

Garnish with a sprig of fresh rosemary or thyme or rose petals, if desired.

Kerchief and Cap
HOT BRANDY

This is your spiced hot brandy for two, and the chamomile tincture lends extra soothing properties. Enjoy in a heatproof mug with a fresh lemon slice and fresh pine sprig for garnish.

Yield: 2 cups, or 2 servings (8 fl oz each)

INGREDIENTS

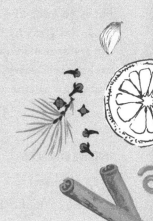

8 fl oz (240 mL) water

8 fl oz (240 mL) cherry shrub

2 cinnamon sticks

6 whole cloves

2 cardamom pods, crushed

2 fresh pine needle sprigs

2 fl oz (60 mL) brandy

2 tsp (10 mL) honey (or other sweetener)

10 drops chamomile tincture

Fresh lemon wheels and fresh pine sprigs for garnish (optional)

DIRECTIONS

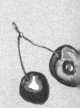

Combine water, cherry shrub, cinnamon sticks, cloves, cardamom pods, and fresh pine needle sprigs in a medium-sized saucepan and bring to a simmer.

Turn heat to low, cover, and let simmer for 12–15 minutes.

Strain the mixture through a fine-mesh sieve, compost herbs, and reserve liquid.

Pour half of the liquid into each of two large heatproof mugs. Add 1 fl oz (30 mL) brandy, 1 tsp (5 mL) honey, and 5 drops chamomile tincture to each mug. Stir to combine.

Garnish each mug with a fresh lemon wheel and pine sprig, if desired.

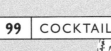

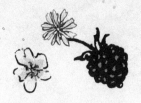

Lung Love Cordial

This pungent herbal cordial is a delicious way to take lung-tonic herbs to keep the respiratory system healthy and hearty. Enjoy in a cordial glass by itself, in a heatproof mug with some hot water for a warm drink, or in a collins glass over ice with some chilled carbonated water, kombucha, or water kefir for a cool drink. Note: this recipe takes 4-6 weeks to prepare.

Yield: 16 fl oz, or 8 servings (2 fl oz each)

INGREDIENTS

1 cup blackberries

8 fl oz (240 mL) brandy

7 tbsp mullein leaf

3 tbsp astragalus root

1 tsp cardamom seed

8 fl oz (240 mL) tulsi syrup

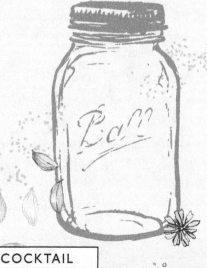

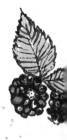

DIRECTIONS

Combine all ingredients in a quart-sized glass jar. Place a piece of natural waxed paper between the jar and lid, cap, and label the jar. Place the jar in a warm, dark location for 4-6 weeks. Invert or roll jar in hands a few times every 1-2 days to mix.

When time is up, strain the mixture through a fine-mesh sieve (lined with an unbleached coffee filter to remove the tiny mullein hairs which can cause irritation), composting the herbs and storing the reserved liquid in a labeled glass jar. Store the cordial in a cool, dark location for up to 1 year (refrigeration is recommended if using a syrup containing less sugar than a 2:1 sugar:water ratio).

To serve, pour 2 fl oz (60 mL) in a cordial glass and sip on its own, add to a heatproof mug of just-boiled water for a quick and easy hot toddy, or add to a collins glass over ice and top with chilled carbonated water, kombucha, or water kefir for a cool, fizzy pick-me-up.

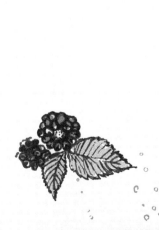
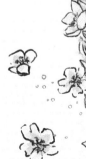
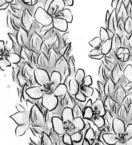

MAITAKE
WHITE RUSSIAN

Make this classic decadent cocktail with a dash of earthiness and the benefits of maitake mushroom—rich in immune-modulating polysaccharides! Enjoy in a rocks glass over ice. Note: the coffee liqueur takes 2-3 weeks to prepare.

INGREDIENTS

2 fl oz (60 mL) vodka

1 fl oz (30 mL) Homemade Coffee Liqueur (ingredients below)

½-1 fl oz (15-30 mL) cream or non-dairy creamer

HOMEMADE COFFEE LIQUEUR:

15 g maitake mushroom or 1 tbsp maitake extract powder

4-8 fl oz (120-240 mL) water

12 fl oz (360 mL) strong hot coffee (regular or decaf)

4 cups (800 g) cane sugar (or sugar alternative)

16 fl oz (480 mL) rum

1 vanilla bean pod

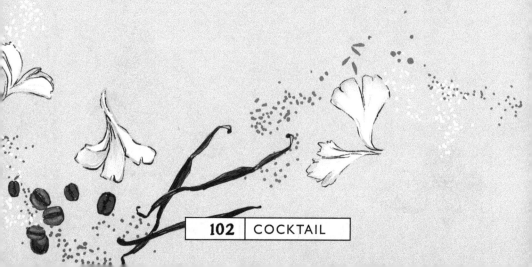

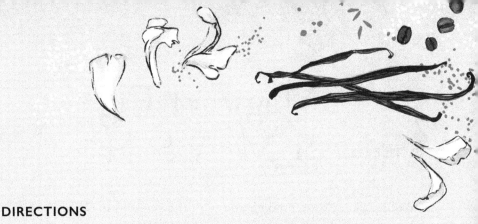

DIRECTIONS

To prepare the coffee liqueur, make a strong decoction by simmering the maitake mushroom in 8 fl oz water, uncovered, until liquid is reduced by half (approximately 4 fl oz (120 mL)). Strain the mixture through a fine-mesh sieve and compost the mushroom pieces. (You can substitute 1 tbsp maitake extract powder mixed with 4 fl oz (120 mL) of hot water for the maitake decoction, if you prefer.)

Combine maitake decoction, hot coffee, and sugar in a quart-sized heat-safe glass canning jar. Stir until sugar is dissolved. Allow to cool to room temperature.

Cut vanilla bean pod in half. Slice the pod lengthwise up the center and using a spoon, scrape the inner flesh out of the pod.

Add rum and vanilla bean inner flesh and cut pod to the mushroom coffee mixture in the glass canning jar. Place a piece of natural waxed paper between the jar and lid, cover, label, and store in a cool, dark location for 2-3 weeks before straining the mixture through a fine-mesh sieve, composting the herbs, and rebottling the liquid in a labeled glass jar. Store in a cool, dark location for up to 1 year.

To prepare the white russian, fill a rocks glass with ice and pour the vodka, coffee liqueur, and cream or non-dairy creamer over the ice. Stir to combine.

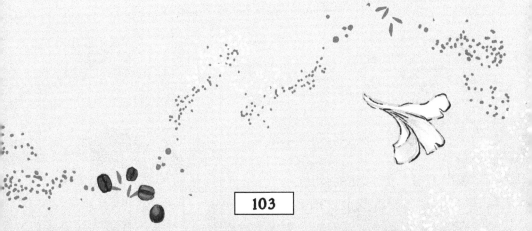

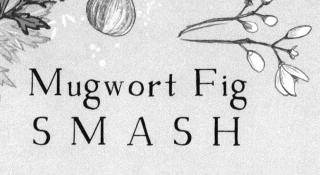

Mugwort Fig
S M A S H

Smoky mugwort scotch combined with the sweetness of fresh figs and a pop of bright orange flavor give this cocktail an enticing flavor that also perks up digestion. Try this unique apéritif for your next fall dinner party! Enjoy in a rocks glass over ice with a fresh fig and an orange twist as a garnish.

INGREDIENTS

2 fl oz (60 mL) mugwort scotch

½ fl oz (15 mL) orange syrup or orange liqueur

4-6 fresh figs, sliced

Fresh fig half and fresh orange twist for garnish (optional)

DIRECTIONS

Fill a rocks glass with ice and set it aside.

Add scotch, figs, and orange syrup to a glass canning jar. Muddle the figs by pressing them against the side of the jar with the back of a spoon.

Fill the jar ⅔ full of ice, cap, and shake hard for 20 seconds. Strain the liquid off the ice and pour it over the ice in the rocks glass.

Garnish with a fresh fig half and orange twist, if desired.

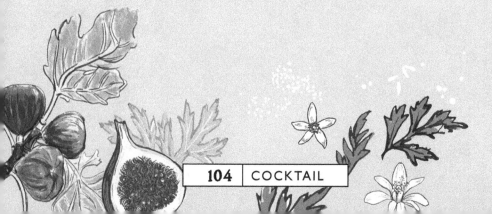

Pear & Ginger *Blitz*

Looking for a simple cocktail full of the flavors of autumn? If so, look no further than this ginger, sage, and pear triplet that will have your guests saying, "Yes, please," at the mere mention of it! Enjoy in a rocks glass over ice with fresh sliced pear as a garnish.

INGREDIENTS

5 fl oz (150 mL) pear juice

1 fl oz (30 mL) ginger vodka

1 fl oz (30 mL) sage syrup

Fresh sliced pear for garnish (optional)

DIRECTIONS

Fill a rocks glass with ice and set it aside.

Combine pear juice, ginger vodka, and sage syrup in a glass canning jar.

Fill the jar ⅔ full of ice, cap, and shake hard for 20 seconds. Strain the liquid off the ice and pour it over the ice in the rocks glass.

Garnish with sliced pear, if desired.

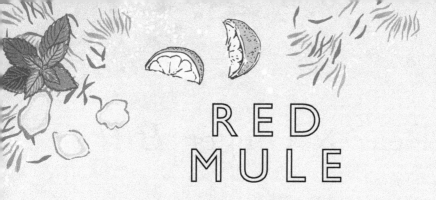

RED MULE

This mixed drink is a botanical twist on the classic mule with its feature of red rooibos, a naturally sweet aromatic South African non-caffeinated tea. Enjoy as a cocktail or mocktail in a rocks glass over ice with a fresh ginger slice or fresh peppermint leaves for garnish.

INGREDIENTS

2 fl oz (60 mL) red rooibos vodka (or cooled red rooibos tea)

1 fl oz (30 mL) ginger syrup

½ fl oz (15 mL) freshly squeezed lime juice

Carbonated water

Fresh ginger slice and a fresh peppermint leaf for garnish (optional)

DIRECTIONS

Fill a rocks glass with ice.

To make a cocktail, combine the red rooibos vodka, ginger syrup, lime juice, and carbonated water in the rocks glass, and stir to combine.

To make a mocktail, combine the red rooibos tea, ginger syrup, lime juice, and carbonated water in the rocks glass, and stir to combine.

Garnish with a slice of fresh ginger and a fresh peppermint leaf, if desired.

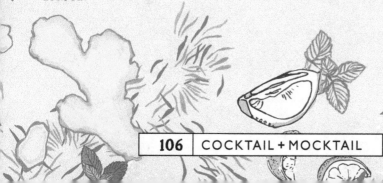

REISHI
Irish Coffee

This is a dark and delectable way to enjoy reishi alongside coffee and whiskey; for a true Irish coffee, be sure to use Irish whiskey, but (shh!) any whiskey will do! Enjoy in a heatproof mug with whipped cream for garnish.

INGREDIENTS

1-2 slices reishi mushroom (or ½ tsp reishi extract powder)

4-8 fl oz (120-240 mL) water

4 fl oz (120 mL) hot coffee (regular or decaf)

1-1½ fl oz (30-45 mL) whiskey

½-1 tbsp (6-12 g) cane sugar (or sugar alternative)

1 fl oz (30 mL) heavy cream (or non-dairy alternative), whipped (optional)

DIRECTIONS

Prepare a strong decoction by combining reishi slices in 8 fl oz water and simmering until liquid is reduced by half (approximately 4 fl oz (120 mL)). Strain and compost the mushroom pieces. (You can substitute ½ tsp reishi extract powder mixed with 4 fl oz (120 mL) of hot water for the reishi decoction, if you prefer.)

Combine the hot reishi decoction, hot coffee, whiskey, and sugar in a heatproof mug.

Top with cream or whipped cream, if desired.

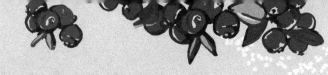

—*Rosehip Cranberry*—
MARGARITA

Instead of the traditional lime juice, this margarita's sour flavor comes from cranberry juice and rosehip, both high in vitamin C. Enjoy this cocktail in a rocks glass over ice with a salt rim and fresh cranberries as a garnish.

INGREDIENTS

2 fl oz (60 mL) tequila

1 fl oz (30 mL) rosehip syrup

1 fl oz (30 mL) unsweetened cranberry juice

Salt for rimming (optional)

Fresh cranberries as a garnish (optional)

DIRECTIONS

Rim a rocks glass with salt, if desired. Carefully fill the glass with ice, being careful not to disturb the salt rim, and set it aside.

Combine tequila, rosehip syrup, and cranberry juice in a glass canning jar.

Fill the jar ⅔ full of ice, cap, and shake hard for 20 seconds. Strain the liquid off the ice and pour it over the ice in the rocks glass, again being careful not to disturb the salt rim.

Garnish with a few fresh cranberries, if desired.

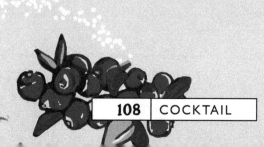

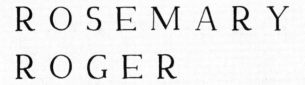
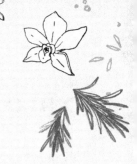

ROSEMARY ROGER

When back-to-school time has you stressing that your brain didn't get quite enough exercise over the summer, whip up this tasty drink for a dose of rosemary and gotu kola, both nootropic and nervine herbs that can help to stimulate cerebral circulation and calm the nervous system. Win, win! Enjoy this cocktail in a collins glass with a fresh orange twist as a garnish.

INGREDIENTS

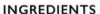

1½ fl oz (45 mL) rosemary rum

½ fl oz (15 mL) apricot brandy

½ fl oz (15 mL) vanilla syrup

3-4 fl oz (90-120 mL) orange juice

1 tsp (5 mL) gotu kola tincture (optional)

Fresh orange twist for garnish (optional)

DIRECTIONS

Fill a collins glass with ice and set it aside.

Place all ingredients, except garnish, in a glass canning jar.

Fill the jar ⅔ full of ice, cap, and shake hard for 20 seconds. Strain the liquid off the ice and pour it over the ice in the collins glass.

Garnish with a fresh orange twist, if desired.

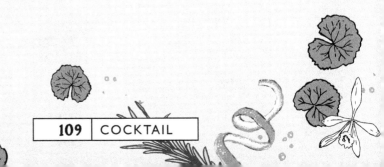

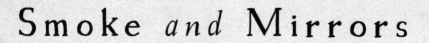

Smoke *and* Mirrors

This may be the perfect autumn drink, especially when paired with a good quality smoky scotch. Infused with dreamy mugwort, this cocktail calls for slow sipping in the evenings while sitting by an open fire and reading a good book. Enjoy in a chilled rocks glass with a piece of candied ginger as a garnish.

INGREDIENTS

2 fl oz (60 mL) mugwort scotch (or plain scotch with 10–15 drops of mugwort tincture)

½–1 fl oz (15–30 mL) ginger syrup

½ fl oz (15 mL) freshly squeezed lemon juice

¼ fl oz (7 mL) smoky single malt scotch

Candied ginger skewer for garnish (optional)

DIRECTIONS

Place a rocks glass in the freezer to chill 30 minutes before serving.

Combine mugwort scotch (or plain scotch with mugwort tincture) with ginger syrup and lemon juice in a glass canning jar.

Fill the jar ⅔ full of ice, cap, and shake hard for 20 seconds. Strain the liquid off the ice and pour it into the chilled rocks glass. Top by pouring the smoky single malt scotch over the top.

Garnish with a candied ginger skewer, if desired.

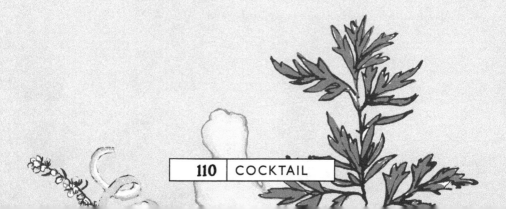

S'more-Tini

Campfires are an autumn must-have and so are the s'mores—
only in liquid form and with a kick of rum and coffee! Enjoy
this cocktail in a martini glass with a graham cracker crumb or
cacao powder rim as a garnish.

INGREDIENTS

1½ fl oz (45 mL) rum

½ fl oz (15 mL) marshmallow root or flower cold-infused tea

¼ fl oz (7 mL) cold brew coffee (regular or decaf) (or roasted
dandelion root coffee)

¾ fl oz (20 mL) cacao nib syrup (made with honey for a honey
graham cracker taste)

½ fl oz (15 mL) heavy cream (or non-dairy alternative)

Honey and crushed graham cracker or cacao powder for rimming
(optional)

DIRECTIONS

Rim a martini glass with honey and crushed graham cracker or
cacao powder, if desired, and set it aside.

Combine rum, marshmallow tea, coffee, cacao nib syrup, and heavy
cream in a glass canning jar.

Fill the jar ⅔ full of ice, cap, and shake hard for 20 seconds.
Strain the liquid off the ice and pour it into the martini glass, being
careful to avoid the graham cracker or cacao powder rim.

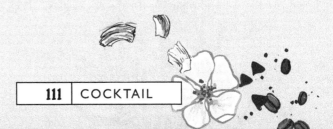

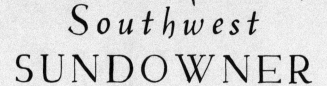

Southwest SUNDOWNER

This relaxing mixed drink features strongly scented and flavorful herbs from hot, dry climates like the Southwest, and it makes a lovely nightcap drink to help settle your body and mind before bed. Enjoy as a cocktail or mocktail in a rocks glass over ice with lavender ice cubes for garnish.

INGREDIENTS

2 fl oz (60 mL) lavender gin (or cooled lavender tea)

½ fl oz (15 mL) juniper syrup

2 fl oz (60 mL) carbonated water

Lavender ice cubes for garnish (optional)

DIRECTIONS

To make lavender ice cubes for garnish, place a few small pieces of fresh or dried lavender in each cavity of an ice cube tray. If using fresh lavender, you can use some of the buds, the fully opened flowers, one or two small pieces of the top of a lavender sprig, or a piece of the stem with some leaves attached. Next, carefully fill each cavity of the tray with water. Don't worry about the lavender floating to the top as this is expected. Place the ice cube tray in the freezer until fully frozen. Add a couple of lavender ice cubes to each drink just before serving for an extra pop of botanical goodness!

Fill a rocks glass with lavender ice cubes, if using, and set it aside.

To make a cocktail, combine the lavender gin and juniper syrup in a glass canning jar.

To make a mocktail, combine the lavender tea and juniper syrup in a glass canning jar.

Fill the jar ⅔ full of ice, cap, and shake hard for 20 seconds. Strain the liquid off the ice and pour it into the rocks glass. Top with carbonated water.

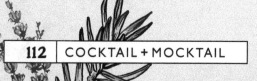

SUMAC 75

The french 75 is a classic mixed drink made with gin, champagne, lemon juice, and sugar and is named after the World War II French 75 mm field gun because drinkers felt it packed a similar punch. However, we're giving it a botanical upgrade with the addition of wild sumac, a sweet and sour berry, and rosehip, both of which offer a hefty vitamin C wallop. Enjoy as a cocktail or mocktail in a champagne flute.

INGREDIENTS

1 fl oz (30 mL) gin (or cooled rose petal tea)

½ fl oz (15 mL) rosehip syrup

½ fl oz (15 mL) sumac cold-infused tea

2 fl oz (60 mL) sparkling rosé wine (or carbonated water)

DIRECTIONS

To make a sumac cold infusion, combine ½ tsp sumac berries with 1 fl oz (30 mL) room temperature water in a mug or jar. Allow this to steep for 1-8 hours in the refrigerator depending on desired flavor before straining through a fine-mesh sieve. Compost or discard the used herbs and reserve ½ fl oz of sumac tea for the recipe.

To make a cocktail, combine the gin, rosehip syrup, and sumac tea in a glass canning jar.

To make a mocktail, combine the rose petal tea, rosehip syrup, and sumac tea in a glass canning jar.

Fill the jar ⅔ full of ice, cap, and shake hard for 20 seconds. Strain the liquid off the ice and pour it into a champagne flute. Top with sparkling rosé wine (for a cocktail) or carbonated water (for a mocktail).

Tulsi Blossom
Spritzer

Serve this spritzer at your next autumn garden party, and you'll be as joyful as the buzzing bees visiting the tulsi patch. Enjoy as a cocktail or mocktail in a wine glass with ice.

INGREDIENTS

2 sprigs fresh tulsi

3 fl oz (90 mL) pinot grigio or other dry white wine (or pear juice or other light fruit juice)

1 fl oz (30 mL) tulsi vodka (or cooled tulsi tea)

½–1 tbsp (7.5–15 mL) honey (or other sweetener)

1 tsp (5 mL) freshly squeezed lemon juice

1–2 fl oz (30–60 mL) carbonated water

Fresh tulsi leaves or sprigs for garnish (optional)

DIRECTIONS

Fill a wine glass with ice and set aside.

Muddle fresh tulsi sprigs in a glass canning jar by pressing them against the side of the jar with the back of a spoon to release their aromatics.

For a cocktail, add wine, tulsi vodka, honey, and lemon juice to the canning jar and mix thoroughly until the honey is dissolved.

For a mocktail, add pear juice, tulsi tea, honey, and lemon juice to the canning jar.

Fill the jar ⅔ full of ice, cap, and shake hard for 20 seconds. Strain the liquid off the ice and pour it over the ice in the wine glass. Top with carbonated water.

Garnish with fresh tulsi leaves or sprigs, if desired.

Tulsi is an utter delight for the senses with its sweet and uplifting scent—it's pure bliss in the late summer garden and in this light and fizzy spritzer—perfect for introducing your guests to this joyful and grounding herb.

JANE METZGER, CO-DIRECTOR OF HERBAL ACADEMY

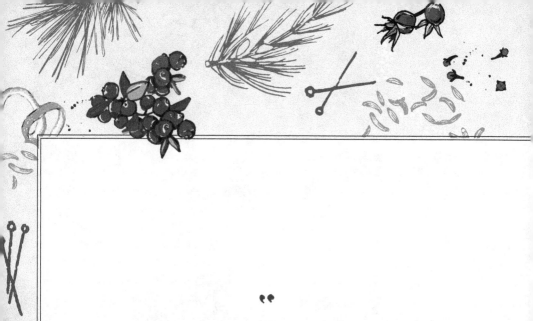

If one takes the time to look, winter can be so breathtakingly beautiful. The bare openness of the landscape is a meditation on stillness and simplicity. Although the air is chill, our hearts are warm when we gather together with family and friends in gratitude.

THE HERBARIUM

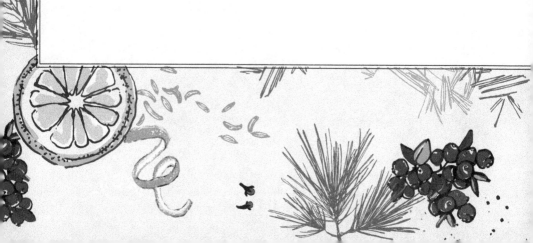

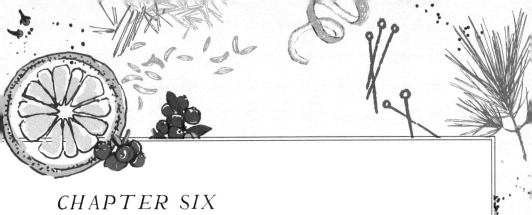

CHAPTER SIX

WINTER BOTANICAL MIXED DRINKS

It's common to feel stagnant during long, cold winter months, which is why many of these botanical mixed drink recipes feature invigorating, warming ingredients, like pepper and pine. These comforting drinks can be sipped solo, or you can be the star of your winter gathering by doubling—or tripling—the recipe to share with friends and loved ones.

While you'll source most of these ingredients from your pantry, foraging for winter ingredients like pine needles or any enduring rose hips is the perfect opportunity to strap on your snow boots and spend an invigorating day outdoors. And when you get home, enjoy a steaming mug of cocoa—or a nip of spiced wine—as a reward for your hard work!

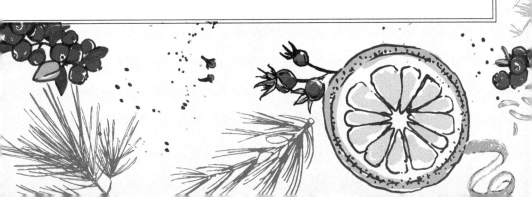

A+ Attention
TONIC

Improve cerebral blood flow and support your memory with this simple mocktail that can help to boost focus and attention. Enjoy warm in a mug or cold in a collins glass, depending on your mood, with a fresh rosemary sprig as a garnish.

INGREDIENTS

4 fl oz (120 mL) carbonated water (or just-boiled water)

2 fl oz (60 mL) A+ Attention Syrup (ingredients below)

½ fl oz (15 mL) freshly squeezed lemon juice

Fresh rosemary sprig for garnish (optional)

A+ ATTENTION SYRUP:

16 fl oz (480 mL) water

8 fl oz (240 mL) honey (or other sweetener)

1 tbsp ginkgo

1 tbsp rosemary

1 tbsp eleuthero

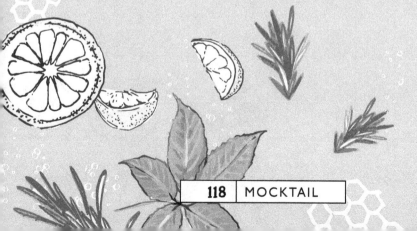

DIRECTIONS

To make the syrup, combine eleuthero and water in a small saucepan. Bring the mixture to a boil and then immediately lower the heat to a simmer. Simmer the mixture until the water level has reduced by half (approximately 8 fl oz (240 mL)). Remove the saucepan from the heat and add ginkgo and rosemary, cover, and allow the mixture to steep until cool. Strain the mixture through a fine-mesh sieve and compost herbs, reserving the finished liquid in a clean bowl. Add the honey (or other sweetener), and stir to thoroughly combine. Transfer the finished syrup to a labeled glass bottle, and store in the refrigerator for up to 2 weeks.

To enjoy warm, add boiled water, syrup, and lemon juice to a heatproof mug, and gently stir to combine.

To enjoy cold, fill a collins glass ⅓ full of ice. Add carbonated water, syrup, and lemon juice to the glass, and gently stir to combine.

Garnish with a fresh rosemary sprig, if desired.

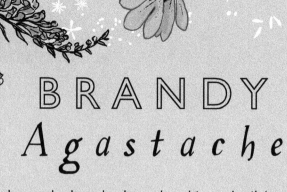

BRANDY
Agastache

An herbal take on the brandy alexander, this cocktail (named for anise hyssop's genus name) is smooth and sweet and chock full of relaxing nervines—try this one at the end of a rough day. Enjoy in a chilled coupe glass.

INGREDIENTS

1 fl oz (30 mL) brandy

½ fl oz (15 mL) rose petal vodka

½ fl oz (15 mL) anise hyssop syrup

1 tsp (5 mL) skullcap tincture

1 fl oz (30 mL) heavy cream (or non-dairy alternative)

DIRECTIONS

Place a coupe glass in the freezer to chill 30 minutes before serving.

Combine all ingredients in a glass canning jar.

Fill the jar ⅔ full of ice, cap, and shake hard for 20 seconds. Strain the liquid off the ice and pour into the chilled coupe glass.

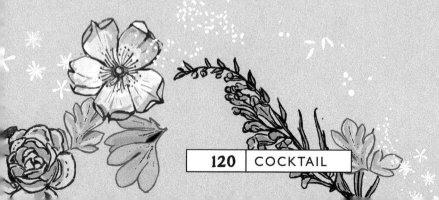

CARDAMOM
Rose EGGNOG

This floral and extra-spicy take on eggnog warms the heart on chilly winter nights. Enjoy this cocktail in a rocks glass with powdered cardamom and a rose petal sugar rim as a garnish.

INGREDIENTS

3 fl oz (90 mL) eggnog (alcohol-free, either homemade or store-bought)

¾ fl oz (20 mL) strong rose petal vodka

1½ fl oz (45 mL) bourbon

½ fl oz (15 mL) cardamom syrup

Powdered cardamom for garnish (optional)

Rose petal sugar for rimming (optional)

DIRECTIONS

Rim a rocks glass in rose petal sugar, if desired, and set it aside.

Combine the remainder of the ingredients, except powdered cardamom, in a glass canning jar.

Fill the jar ⅔ full of ice, cap, and shake hard for 20 seconds. Strain the liquid off the ice and pour into the rocks glass, being careful not to disturb the rose petal sugar rim.

Garnish with powdered cardamom, if desired.

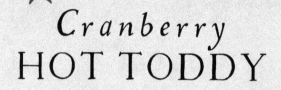

Cranberry
HOT TODDY

Cozy up on a cold winter's day with something warm and festive—something that also includes an extra boost of wellness benefits! This winter hot toddy cocktail checks all the boxes with festive and vitamin C-rich cranberry and warming, antimicrobial spices. Enjoy this cocktail in a heatproof mug.

Yield: 36 fl oz, or 6 servings (6 fl oz each)

INGREDIENTS

30 fl oz (900 mL) pure cranberry juice

⅓–½ cup (67–100 g) cane sugar (or sugar alternative)

1 tsp whole allspice

2 cinnamon sticks

1-inch piece fresh ginger, sliced

½ tsp whole cloves (adjust to taste)

2 star anise pods (optional)

6 fl oz (180 mL) dark liquor (rum, whiskey, or bourbon)

DIRECTIONS

Add cranberry juice, sugar, allspice, cinnamon sticks, ginger, cloves, and star anise to a large saucepan and bring to a boil. Immediately reduce to a simmer, stirring to dissolve sugar.

Cover and simmer on low for about 10 minutes. Reduce heat and keep warm until ready to serve.

When ready to serve, carefully strain the mixture through a fine-mesh sieve, composting the herbs and reserving the liquid. Add the liquor to the reserved cranberry spice liquid, stir once more, and divide into individual heatproof mugs.

Evergreen
HIGHBALL

The uplifting and warming nature of pine combined with the floral sweetness of anise hyssop makes this highball a comforting winter pick-me-up that doubles as a perfect after-dinner digestif—both pine and anise hyssop have carminative properties and help encourage digestion after those heavy winter meals. Enjoy this cocktail in a collins glass over ice with a fresh pine sprig as a garnish.

INGREDIENTS

2 fl oz (60 mL) bourbon

¾ fl oz (20 mL) pine syrup

½ fl oz (15 mL) anise hyssop syrup

5 fl oz (150 mL) carbonated water

Fresh pine sprig for garnish (optional)

DIRECTIONS

Fill a collins glass with ice and set it aside.

Combine bourbon, pine syrup, and anise hyssop syrup in a glass canning jar.

Fill the jar ⅔ full of ice, cap, and shake hard for 20 seconds. Strain the liquid off the ice and pour over the ice in the collins glass. Top with carbonated water and gently stir to combine.

Garnish with a fresh pine sprig, if desired.

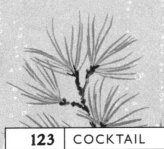

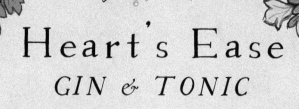

Heart's Ease
GIN & TONIC

Rose and hawthorn have long been used to uplift the spirit, ease grief, and bring comfort to the heart. This duo is combined for a heart-happy take on the classic gin and tonic. Enjoy in a collins glass over ice with rose petals as a garnish.

INGREDIENTS

2 fl oz (60 mL) rose petal gin

1 fl oz (30 mL) hawthorn berry syrup

4 fl oz (120 mL) tonic water (or carbonated water)

Rose petals for garnish (optional)

DIRECTIONS

Fill a collins glass with ice.

Layer rose petal gin, hawthorn berry syrup, and tonic water (or carbonated water) over the ice, and give the drink a gentle stir before serving.

Garnish with rose petals, if desired.

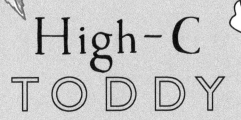

High-C
TODDY

The cold, dark days of winter can feel neverending, but sipping an occasional cup of this high-C toddy can help to dispel any gloomy moods. Packed with vitamin C-rich herbs, it's a great way to support your immune system during the cold and flu season as well! Enjoy as a cocktail or mocktail in your favorite heatproof mug with a fresh lemon slice for garnish.

INGREDIENTS

2 fl oz (60 mL) whiskey (or black tea)

½ fl oz (15 mL) rosehip syrup

½ fl oz (15 mL) sumac syrup

½ fl oz (15 mL) ginger syrup

½ fl oz (15 mL) freshly squeezed lemon juice

Boiling water

Fresh lemon slice for garnish (optional)

DIRECTIONS

To make a cocktail, combine the whiskey, syrups, and lemon juice in a heatproof mug. Top with boiling water and stir.

To make a mocktail, brew a cup of black tea and add the syrups and lemon juice to it in a heatproof mug.

Garnish with a lemon slice, if desired.

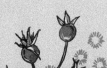

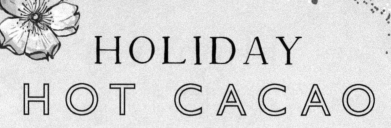

HOLIDAY
HOT CACAO

Put yourself (or guests) in the holiday spirit with this red rose and green peppermint hot chocolate recipe! This festive minty hot cacao recipe serves up beautifully and can be enjoyed by yourself or with a group. Enjoy in a heatproof mug with a dollop of whipped cream, chocolate shavings, and crushed rose petals as a garnish.

INGREDIENTS

8 fl oz (240 mL) milk of choice (dairy or non-dairy)

1 tbsp peppermint leaf

1 tbsp cacao powder

1 fl oz (30 mL) rose petal syrup

Whipped cream, chocolate shavings, and crushed rose petals for garnish (optional)

DIRECTIONS

Place peppermint leaf and milk in a saucepan and bring to a simmer over low heat. As soon as the mixture begins to steam, remove the saucepan from the heat, cover with a lid, and allow it to steep for 10 minutes.

After 10 minutes, carefully strain the mixture through a fine-mesh sieve, composting the peppermint leaves. Whisk in the cacao powder and rose petal syrup until the mixture is smooth. Serve immediately in a heatproof mug or return to heat if the mixture needs to be warmed.

Garnish with a dollop of whipped cream sprinkled with chocolate shavings and crushed rose petals, if desired.

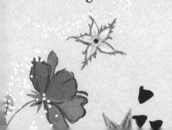

"

Holiday Hot Cacao is like sweet wintery, minty herbal cheer in a mug & best enjoyed with loved ones and heartfelt conversation.

AMBER MEYERS, CO-DIRECTOR OF HERBAL ACADEMY

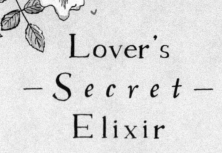
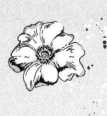

Lover's
— S e c r e t —
Elixir

This tasty aphrodisiac elixir is so yummy that it can be added to drinks and desserts in such a way that your lover won't even know it's there to serve a purpose! This herbal combination helps to soothe emotions while stimulating blood flow and supporting the heart simultaneously. Enjoy this elixir in your favorite cocktail, over dessert, or on its own by the spoonful. Ginseng may be stimulating so this elixir may be best avoided prior to bedtime. Note: this recipe takes 1 week to prepare.

Yield: 5 fl oz, or 30 servings (1 tsp each)

INGREDIENTS

1 fl oz (30 mL) Chocolate Ginseng Decoction (ingredients below)

⅓ cup (67 g) cane sugar (or sugar alternative)

2½ fl oz (75 mL) boiling water

1½ fl oz (45 mL) rose petal gin

1 tsp (5 mL) vanilla extract

CHOCOLATE GINSENG DECOCTION:

1 tsp cacao nibs

1 tsp ginseng (sustainably cultivated source only)

1 tsp rose petal

2 fl oz (60 mL) water

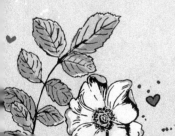

DIRECTIONS

Combine cacao nibs, ginseng, and water in a small saucepan. Bring to a boil over medium heat and immediately turn the heat down to low to let the mixture simmer until the water has reduced by half (approximately 1 fl oz (30 mL)). Remove from heat, add rose petals, cover, and let steep for 10 minutes. After 10 minutes, strain the mixture through a fine-mesh sieve. Compost the herbs and reserve the warm liquid in a quart-sized glass canning jar.

Add sugar and boiling water to the chocolate ginseng decoction, stirring continually, until the sugar is dissolved and the mixture is thoroughly combined. Set aside to cool.

Once cool, add rose petal gin and vanilla extract and stir to combine. Transfer elixir to a labeled glass jar and store in the refrigerator for 1 week before using. Use within 2-3 weeks.

To serve, add 1 tsp to a cocktail, drizzle over a dessert, or enjoy on its own, as desired.

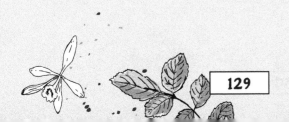

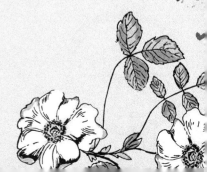

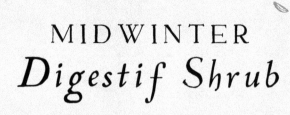

MIDWINTER
Digestif Shrub

A little sweet and a little sour, this flavor-packed shrub is a perfect drink to sip slowly after a hearty winter meal. Formulated with botanicals that help support digestion and ease gas, bloating, and cramping, this winter shrub mocktail will also warm you from the inside out if you're feeling a bit chilly. Enjoy in a rocks glass.

INGREDIENTS

½ fl oz (15 mL) orange syrup

½ fl oz (15 mL) fennel syrup

¼ fl oz (7 mL) clove syrup

½–1½ tsp (2.5–7.5 mL) chamomile vinegar (to taste)

4 fl oz (120 mL) carbonated water, chilled

DIRECTIONS

Combine syrups and vinegar in a rocks glass. Top with chilled carbonated water and gently stir to combine.

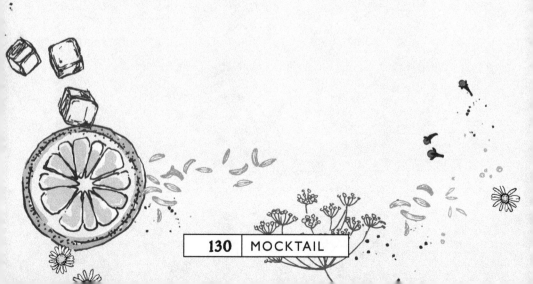

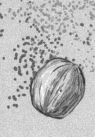

MIGHTY MUSHROOM
Cocoa Latte

Warm up with a cozy mushroom cocoa latte. This one is mighty in adaptogenic, immune-boosting mushrooms, and a cozy drink to sip all winter long. Enjoy in a heatproof mug with cacao nibs and powdered cinnamon as a garnish.

INGREDIENTS

12 fl oz (360 mL) milk of choice (dairy or non-dairy)

1 tsp reishi mushroom extract powder

1 tsp cordyceps mushroom extract powder

2 tsp (10 mL) maple syrup

1 tsp almond butter

1½ tsp cacao powder

1 pinch nutmeg powder

1 pinch cardamom powder

1 pinch cinnamon powder

1 pinch sea salt

Cacao nibs and powdered cinnamon for garnish (optional)

DIRECTIONS

Place mushroom powders, maple syrup, almond butter, cacao powder, nutmeg, cardamom, cinnamon, and sea salt in a small blender.

Heat the milk of choice until hot, then pour into the blender. Blend on high for approximately 30 seconds or until slightly frothy.

Pour the latte into a heatproof mug.

Garnish with a sprinkle of cacao nibs and a dash of powdered cinnamon, if desired.

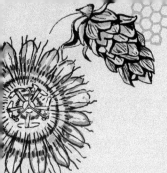
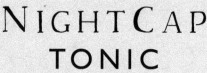

NIGHTCAP
TONIC

Tinctures blend beautifully into cocktails and offer nearly endless combinations. This bedtime tonic combines a few sleepy-time tinctures, including hops, passionflower, and valerian, with honey and brandy for an easy-to-make cocktail intended to help you drift to sleep. Enjoy in a cordial glass.

INGREDIENTS

1 fl oz (30 mL) brandy

1 tsp (5 mL) NightCap Syrup (ingredients below)

NIGHTCAP SYRUP:

4 fl oz (120 mL) honey (or other sweetener)

1 fl oz (30 mL) hops tincture

1 fl oz (30 mL) passionflower tincture

1 fl oz (30 mL) valerian tincture

1 fl oz (30 mL) chamomile tincture

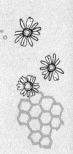

DIRECTIONS

To make the nightcap syrup, thoroughly mix honey and tinctures together until well combined. Transfer the mixture to a labeled glass jar and store in a cool, dark location for up to 1 year.

To mix the drink, combine 1 fl oz of brandy with 1 tsp of nightcap syrup in a cordial glass. Stir until well combined, and sip slowly as you prepare to blissfully drift to sleep.

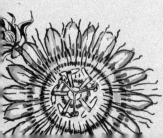
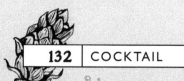

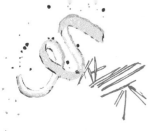

PEPPER + PINE

Feeling a bit slow and sluggish? Put a little pep in your step with this zingy combination of pepper and pine, where hints of citrus, conifer, and spice all mingle in your mouth together. Enjoy as a cocktail or mocktail in a chilled martini glass with a fresh lemon twist as a garnish.

INGREDIENTS

2 fl oz (60 mL) pine gin (or cooled pine tea)

1 fl oz (30 mL) black pepper syrup

½ fl oz (15 mL) freshly squeezed lemon juice

Fresh lemon twist for garnish (optional)

DIRECTIONS

Place a martini glass in the freezer to chill 30 minutes before serving.

To make a cocktail, combine the pine gin, black pepper syrup, and lemon juice in a glass canning jar.

To make a mocktail, combine the pine tea, black pepper syrup, and lemon juice in a glass canning jar.

Fill the jar ⅔ full of ice, cap, and shake hard for 20 seconds. Strain the liquid off the ice and pour into a chilled martini glass.

Garnish with a fresh lemon twist, if desired.

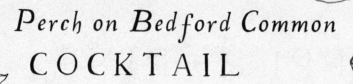

Perch on Bedford Common
COCKTAIL

Perch on Bedford Common is the home of Herbal Academy's schoolhouse! This recipe is inspired by the Bedford, a cocktail created by Del Pedro at Grange Hall in New York's West Village. Both the ashwagandha and chamomile are added for their relaxing effects. Enjoy in a rocks glass with a fresh orange slice or mint sprig as a garnish.

INGREDIENTS

2 fl oz (60 mL) apple shrub

1 fl oz (30 mL) rye whiskey

2 tsp (10 mL) sweet vermouth

1 tsp (5 mL) orange liqueur

1 tsp (5 mL) vanilla syrup

10 drops ashwagandha tincture

2 dashes (20 drops) chamomile bitters

Orange slice or fresh mint sprig for garnish (optional)

DIRECTIONS

Fill a rocks glass with ice and set it aside.

Combine the apple shrub, rye whiskey, sweet vermouth, orange liqueur, vanilla syrup, and ashwagandha tincture in a glass canning jar.

Fill the jar ⅔ full of ice, cap, and shake hard for 20 seconds. Strain the liquid off the ice and pour over the ice in the rocks glass. Top with chamomile bitters.

Garnish with a fresh orange slice or a fresh mint sprig, if desired.

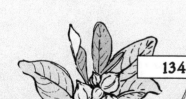

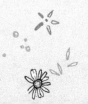

ROSEMARY CITRUS
OLD FASHIONED

This herb-and-fruit cocktail concoction is a spin on a classic old fashioned, combining notes of astringency with bright and aromatic flavors. As a bonus, rosemary promotes mental clarity and memory capabilities. Enjoy in a rocks glass with a fresh rosemary sprig.

INGREDIENTS

2 fl oz (60 mL) rosemary bourbon

1 fl oz (30 mL) orange syrup

½ fl oz (15 mL) freshly squeezed lemon juice

½ tsp (2.5 mL) orange bitters

2 fl oz (60 mL) carbonated water, chilled

Fresh rosemary sprig for garnish (optional)

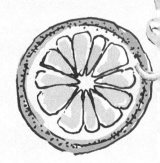

DIRECTIONS

Fill a rocks glass with ice and set it aside.

Combine rosemary bourbon, orange syrup, lemon juice, and orange bitters in a glass canning jar.

Fill the jar ⅔ full of ice, cap, and shake hard for 20 seconds. Strain the liquid off the ice and pour over the ice in the rocks glass. Top with chilled carbonated water.

Garnish with a fresh rosemary sprig, if desired.

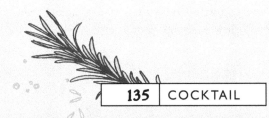

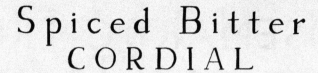

Spiced Bitter
CORDIAL

With bitter angelica and the addition of warming spices, this bitter cordial recipe is great for digestive support during the cold, dark winter months. Enjoy in a cordial glass by itself, in a heatproof mug with some hot water for a warm drink, or in a collins class with some carbonated water, kombucha, or water kefir for a cool drink. Note: this recipe takes 4-6 weeks to prepare.

Yield: 36 fl oz, or 18 servings (2 fl oz each)

INGREDIENTS

1 cup angelica root

⅓ cup cinnamon sticks, crushed

¼ cup fresh ginger, minced

⅛ cup whole cloves

⅛ cup cardamom pod, crushed

32 fl oz (960 mL) gin

8 fl oz (240 mL) honey (or other sweetener)

DIRECTIONS

Combine all ingredients in a quart-sized glass jar. Place a piece of natural waxed paper between the jar and lid, cap, and label the jar. Place the jar in a warm, dark location for 4-6 weeks. Invert or roll jar in hands a few times every 1-2 days to mix.

When time is up, strain the mixture through a fine-mesh sieve, composting the herbs and storing the reserved liquid in a labeled glass jar. Store in a cool, dark location for 1-2 years.

To serve, pour 2 fl oz (60 mL) in a cordial glass and sip on its own, add to a heatproof mug of just-boiled water for a quick and easy hot toddy, or add to a collins glass and top with carbonated water, kombucha, or water kefir for a cool, fizzy pick-me-up.

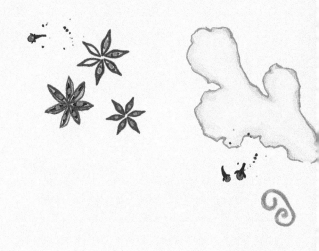

The bare silhouettes of trees offer a dramatic sight against the pale skies of winter. Bearing witness to the turning of the seasons can be a profound experience throughout the year, but winter's stark beauty brings a special sense of stillness that invites moments of pause and reflection.

THE HERBARIUM

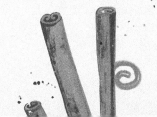

Sweet Spiced Wine

Elevate your next holiday gathering with this botanical spiced wine recipe. It's warming, flavorful, and fragrant, filled with botanicals that support the immune system, and it will take the cozy factor of your gathering to the next level! Enjoy in a heatproof mug with fresh orange slices, cranberries, or dried cinnamon sticks as a garnish.

Yield: 24 fl oz, or 4 servings (6 fl oz each)

INGREDIENTS

1 bottle (750 mL) fruity red wine

½–1 fl oz (15–30 mL) elderberry or rosehip syrup

1 fresh orange

½ cup fresh cranberries

6 whole cloves

2 cinnamon sticks

3 star anise pods

Fresh orange slices, cranberries, or dried cinnamon sticks for garnish (optional)

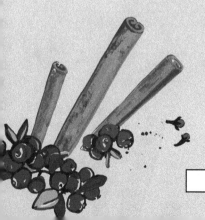

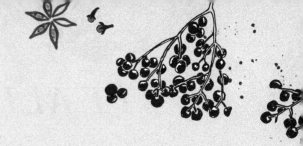

DIRECTIONS

Begin by cutting an orange in half. Squeeze the juice from one half of the orange into a saucepan and slice the other half, adding the slices to the saucepan.

Next, add all of the other ingredients, except for garnishes, to the saucepan. Begin with only ½ fl oz of elderberry or rosehip syrup as you can always add more later, to taste. Heat the mixture over medium heat until it begins to steam. At that point, turn the heat to low and allow the mixture to steep for 20 minutes, covered.

Carefully taste the mixture to see if it's sweet and spicy enough for you. If you want to add the remaining elderberry or rosehip syrup, feel free to do so now. Keep in mind that the longer you simmer the mixture, the spicier it will taste.

If you're happy with the flavor, serve now or keep on low heat, covered, to keep the mixture warm until you're ready to serve.

Pour into individual heatproof mugs and garnish with extra orange slices, cranberries, or cinnamon sticks, if desired.

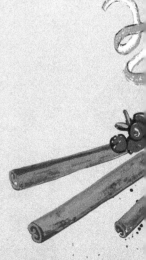

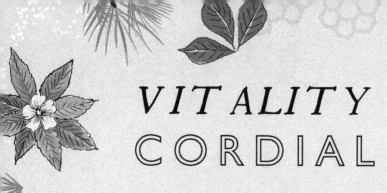

VITALITY
CORDIAL

This cordial recipe uses fresh conifer needles and other botanicals that promote longevity. It is designed to build strength and vitality in the body and is particularly useful during the long, cold, dark days of the winter season. Enjoy in a cordial glass by itself, in a heatproof mug with some hot water for a warm drink, or in a collins class with some carbonated water, kombucha, or water kefir for a cool drink. Ginseng may be stimulating so this cordial may be best avoided prior to bedtime. Note: this recipe takes 4-6 weeks to prepare.

Yield: 30 fl oz, or 15 servings (2 fl oz each)

INGREDIENTS

1 oz pine needle or spruce tips, chopped

½ oz damiana

½ oz ginseng (sustainably sourced only)

16 fl oz (480 mL) brandy (or enough to fill jar)

8 fl oz (240 mL) honey (or other sweetener)

8 fl oz (240 mL) water

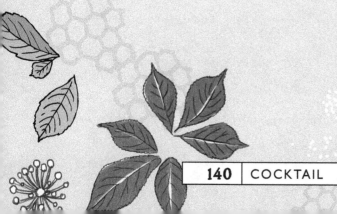

DIRECTIONS

Note that spruce tips are the tender new spring growth of spruce, and these are a great option if making this recipe in the spring. Otherwise, pine needle, which is available year-round, even in the winter, is a good option.

Combine all ingredients in a quart-sized glass jar. Place a piece of natural waxed paper between the jar and lid, cap, and label the jar. Place the jar in a warm, dark location for 4-6 weeks. Invert or roll jar in hands a few times every 1-2 days to mix.

When time is up, strain the mixture through a fine-mesh sieve, composting the herbs and storing the reserved liquid in a labeled glass jar. Store in a cool, dark location for up to 1 year.

To serve, pour 2 fl oz (60 mL) in a cordial glass and sip on its own, add to a heatproof mug of just-boiled water for a quick and easy hot toddy, or add to a collins glass and top with carbonated water, kombucha, or water kefir for a cool, fizzy pick-me-up.

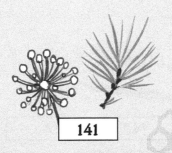

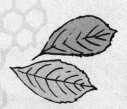

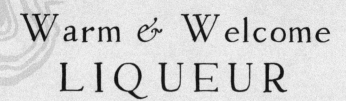

Warm & Welcome
LIQUEUR

This tasty liqueur is a sensual sipping elixir that's both pleasurable, gently stimulating, and warming to the whole body. It makes a nice gift or can be enjoyed on a cold winter's evening, perhaps reserved just for you and your loved one. Enjoy in a cordial glass by itself, in a heatproof mug with some hot water for a warm drink, or in a collins class with some carbonated water, kombucha, or water kefir for a cool drink. Note: this recipe takes 5-9 weeks to prepare.

Yield: 22 fl oz, or 11 servings (2 fl oz each)

INGREDIENTS

2 vanilla bean pods

2 cinnamon sticks

½ oz damiana

2 tbsp pecans (optional)

16 fl oz (480 mL) bourbon

8 fl oz (240 mL) honey (or other sweetener)

Cinnamon powder (optional)

Vanilla extract (optional)

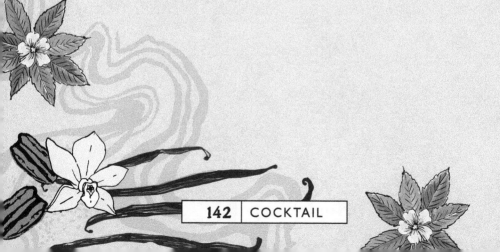

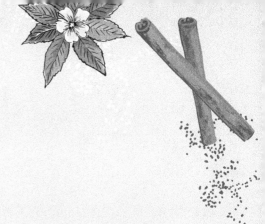

DIRECTIONS

Cut vanilla bean pods in half. Slice each pod lengthwise up the center and using a spoon, scrape the inner flesh out of the pod. Place the inner flesh and cut pods in a quart-sized glass canning jar.

Combine the remaining ingredients in the glass canning jar along with the vanilla bean pods. Place a piece of natural waxed paper between the jar and the lid and seal. Label and place in a warm, dark location to infuse for 1-2 weeks for a mild flavor and 2-4 weeks for a stronger flavor. Invert or roll jar in hands a few times every 1-2 days to mix.

When time is up, strain the mixture through a fine-mesh sieve. Compost the herbs and transfer the liquid to a clean labeled glass jar. Using a clean spoon, taste the liquid and adjust flavors if needed. Feel free to add some vanilla extract to enhance the vanilla flavor, or some cinnamon powder to increase the cinnamon flavor.

Once you are happy with the flavor, store the mixture in a cool, dark location for 1 month to allow the flavors to mellow and smooth before consuming. Use completely within 1-2 years.

To serve, pour 2 fl oz (60 mL) in a cordial glass and sip on its own, add to a heatproof mug of just-boiled water for a quick and easy hot toddy, or add to a collins glass and top with carbonated water, kombucha, or water kefir for a cool, fizzy pick-me-up.

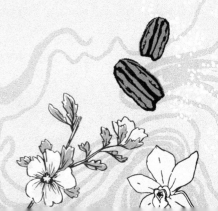

Woodland
GIMLET

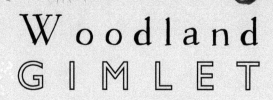

A gimlet is a light cocktail usually found on brunch menus but can be enjoyed any time of the day or on any occasion. This particular gimlet recipe is filled with woodland scents and flavors and is perfect for outdoor celebrations. Enjoy as a cocktail or mocktail in a rocks glass over ice with a fresh lime twist and pine sprig for garnish.

INGREDIENTS

2 fl oz (60 mL) pine gin (or cooled pine tea)

1 fl oz (30 mL) rosemary syrup

½ fl oz (15 mL) freshly squeezed lime juice

10 drops wild cherry bark tincture (or wild cherry bark vinegar)

Fresh lime twist and pine sprig for garnish (optional)

DIRECTIONS

Fill a rocks glass with ice and set it aside.

To make a cocktail, combine the pine gin, rosemary syrup, lime juice, and wild cherry bark tincture in a glass canning jar.

To make a mocktail, combine the pine tea, rosemary syrup, lime juice, and wild cherry bark vinegar in a glass canning jar.

Fill the jar ⅔ full of ice, cap, and shake hard for 20 seconds. Strain the liquid off the ice and pour over the ice in the rocks glass.

Garnish with a fresh lime twist and a pine sprig, if desired.

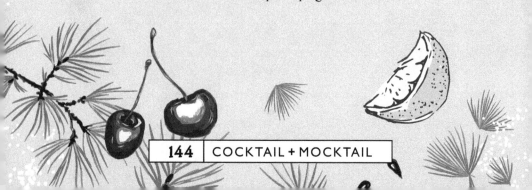

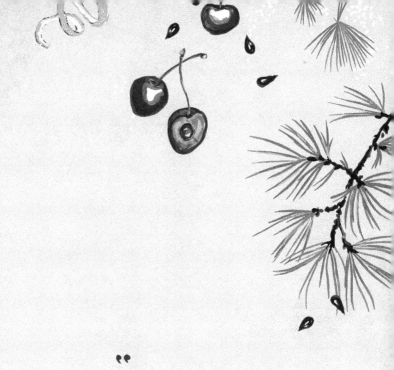

‚‚

There is nothing so refreshing as the flavor of conifer in the winter. and the Woodland Gimlet certainly delivers. It adds just enough of the evergreen essence you expect during the season. while at the same time. a touch of fresh crispness that gives you hope for the coming spring.

MEAGAN VISSER, BSN, STAFF HERBALIST AT HERBAL ACADEMY

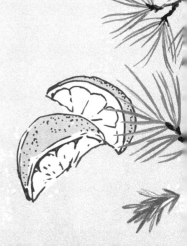

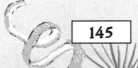

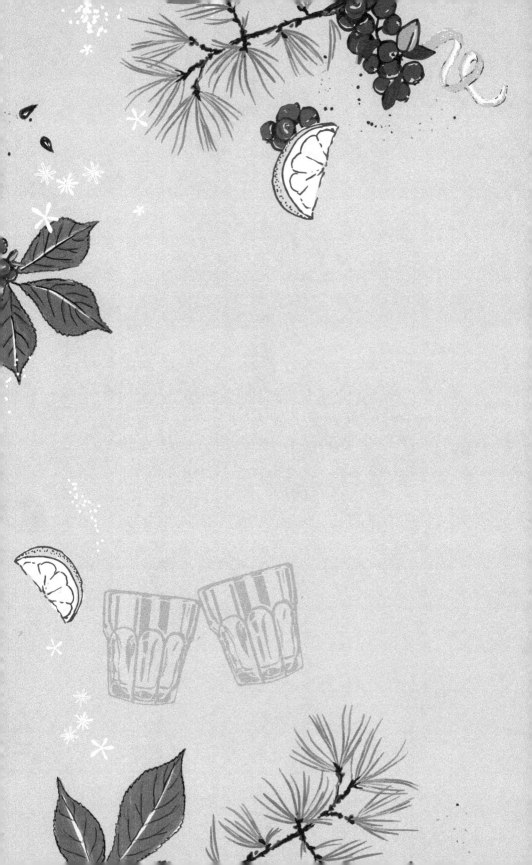

A TOAST TO YOU!

Thank you for joining us in the art of herbal mixology and the adventures that come with this Botanical Mixed Drinks Recipe Book!

As we moved through the seasons together—filling our cups with vibrant and seasonal mixed drinks—we hope you learned a bit more about yourself. Are you a down-to-earth forager who enjoys trekking through the woods to uncover the ingredients for a rooty beverage with burdock and dandelion? Or are you more of an elevated sipper—blending your bubbly champagne with delicate rose and fresh strawberries? Perhaps you're a little bit of both, depending on the day and your mood.

As you muddled herbs, mixed syrups, and poured bitters, you may have felt a spark that all of us at the Herbal Academy have in common—the flickering desire to learn more about the ancient and time-tested world of herbs. If you're kindling that spark now, then this book can serve as your gateway to learning how to use herbs in every aspect of your home—from your kitchen to your wellness cabinet, and so much more.

At the Herbal Academy, we teach budding and experienced herbalists how to make safe, effective, and delicious recipes that unlock the supportive power of herbs and spices. We offer dozens of online courses, workshops, and intensives on a variety of herb-related topics. You can explore more mixology magic in our **Botanical Mixed Drinks Workshop**, which inspired this book, dive even deeper into herbal drinks by enrolling in **The Craft of Herbal Fermentation Course,** or get started with blending your own herbal

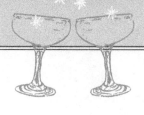

teas in the **Tea Blending 101 Workshop**. If you would like to learn more about foraging for botanicals, then join us in **The Foraging Course** or the **Botany & Wildcrafting Course**—both of which share how to safely and sustainably identify, harvest, and use the plants that are native to your region. Or perhaps you're ready for a well-rounded, in-depth herbal education that explores the supportive properties of dozens of different herbs—and how to transform those herbs into nourishing edible and topical recipes, from tinctures and teas to oils and salves—which is what you'll find in our **Introductory Herbal Course**.

Explore all of our courses and workshops at *theherbalacademy.com*

an HERBAL COMMUNITY

We're blessed to be a part of a vibrant community of herbalists, gardeners, foragers, and botanically inspired folks. We'd love to connect with you personally and cheer you on as you bring these botanical mixed drink recipes to life. We invite you to share the recipes you make with us on social media by tagging us in your post or using the hashtag #myherbalstudies. We can't wait to see what you make!

Cheers from your friends and educators at the Herbal Academy!

INSTAGRAM
@herbalacademy

FACEBOOK
@theherbalacademy

PINTEREST
@theherbalacademy

YOUTUBE
@herbalacademy

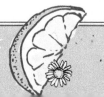

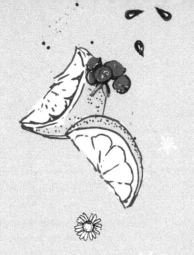

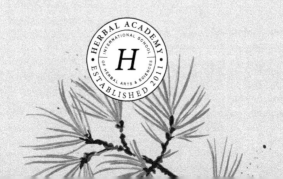

INDEX

INDEX OF RECIPES BY TYPE

INDEX OF RECIPES BY SEASON

INDEX OF RECIPES BY HERB

153

INDEX OF RECIPES BY ALCOHOL TYPE

EXPAND YOUR HERBAL LIBRARY
with the Herbal Academy's complete Recipe Book Collection!

BOTANICAL SKIN CARE RECIPE BOOK

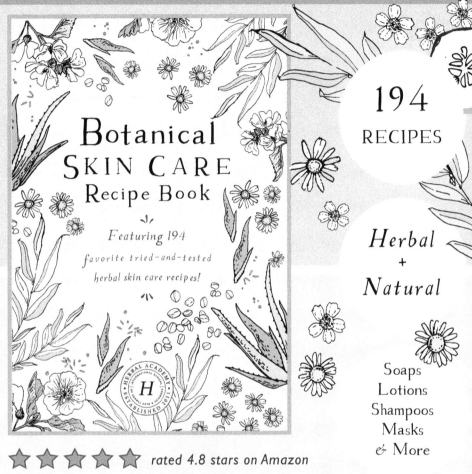

194 RECIPES

Herbal + Natural

Soaps
Lotions
Shampoos
Masks
& More

⭐⭐⭐⭐⭐ rated 4.8 stars on Amazon

If you loved the **Botanical Mixed Drinks Recipe Book**, you're in for another treat with the **Botanical Skin Care Recipe Book**—the first installment in the Herbal Academy's inspiring Recipe Book Collection! Expand your herbal skills and compendium with 194 tried-and-tested, herbalist-approved body-care recipes using herbs and natural ingredients you will actually want to put on your skin and body.

Curated by the Herbal Academy's trusted team of herbalists and formulators with a 4.8 rating by readers, this popular recipe book will help build your confidence making safe and effective skin-care products with preparations that are well loved and well used.

If you want to fill your cupboard with incredible botanical skin-care products, shop this recipe book alongside other herbal books and textbooks on the Herbal Academy's website:

WWW.THEHERBALACADEMY.COM/SHOP

CPSIA information can be obtained
at www.ICGtesting.com
Printed in the USA
JSHW011639120323
38819JS00006B/14